Urbanization and its implications for child health

Potential for action

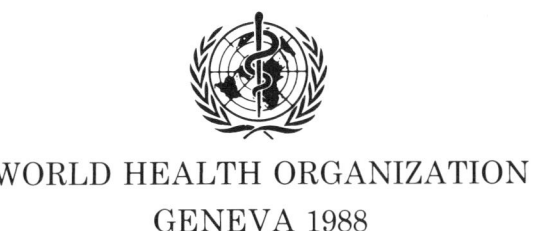

WORLD HEALTH ORGANIZATION
GENEVA 1988

ISBN 92 4 156123 8

© World Health Organization, 1988

Publications of the World Health Organization enjoy copyright protection in accordance with the provisions of Protocol 2 of the Universal Copyright Convention. For rights of reproduction or translation of WHO publications, in part or *in toto*, application should be made to the Office of Publications, World Health Organization, Geneva, Switzerland. The World Health Organization welcomes such applications.

The designations employed and the presentation of the material in this publication do not imply the expression of any opinion whatsoever on the part of the Secretariat of the World Health Organization concerning the legal status of any country, territory, city or area or of its authorities, or concerning the delimitation of its frontiers or boundaries.

The mention of specific companies or of certain manufacturers' products does not imply that they are endorsed or recommended by the World Health Organization in preference to others of a similar nature that are not mentioned. Errors and omissions excepted, the names of proprietary products are distinguished by initial capital letters.

TYPESET IN INDIA
PRINTED IN ENGLAND
88/7616—Macmillan/Clays—5000

Contents

Preface v

Acknowledgements vi

Introduction 1
The gap between needs and responses 2
The lack of resources 5

1. Living conditions and health problems in urban centres 9
Background—the global picture 9
Water and sanitation 15
Air and water pollution 17
Health hazards of poverty 18

2. Housing and health 32
Background 32
How the urban poor find somewhere to live 37

3. Neighbourhood organizations and health 44
How and why neighbourhood organizations are formed 44
Three case studies from Latin America 46

4. The role of local government 50
Local government and health 50
Local government and neighbourhood associations 52
Confronting the problem as a whole 56

5. Summary, conclusions, and recommendations 63
Targeting services and support to those most in need 64
Coordination of action 65
The key role of local government 69
The role of nongovernmental organizations 70
National government 70
Aid agencies 72

References   74

Annex 1. WHO/UNEP Technical Panel on Environmental Health Aspects of Housing and Urban Planning   79

Preface

The World Health Organization (WHO) and the United Nations Environment Programme (UNEP) are striving to ensure the inclusion of environmental health measures in the planning and development of human settlements. This task involves the provision of information about current conditions and trends, and the preparation of environmental health criteria and guidelines. Material of this nature is useful to decision-makers and professional personnel, not only in the health sector, but in such sectors as housing, public works, and socioeconomic planning.

The present book explores trends in urbanization, the effect of these trends on the physical and social environment of urban settlements, and the impact of this environment on child health. The measures taken by certain governments and experience to date of community participation in tackling the problems of urban growth have provided valuable insights into possibilities for future action. It is hoped that this publication will help to increase awareness of the severe and pervasive impact on health of the deteriorating environmental conditions produced by too rapid urbanization, and that it will promote widespread consideration of policies and action that could improve the situation.

The idea for this publication arose from discussions between representatives of the United Nations Centre for Human Settlements (UNCHS), UNEP and WHO, which highlighted the need for new and improved ways of dealing with environmental conditions in low-income settlements. A WHO/UNEP Technical Panel on Environmental Health Aspects of Housing and Urban Planning which met in Moscow, USSR, in April 1985 selected this topic, *inter alia*, for priority preparation as an information and guideline document. The Panel also drew up a proposed outline for this publication, including statements on background, needs, technical content, format, and expected impact. A list of the participants will be found in Annex 1.

Acknowledgements

WHO wishes to express its appreciation to the staff of the Latin American office of the International Institute for Environment and Development and the Centre for Urban and Regional Studies, Buenos Aires, who undertook the preparation of the first draft of this document. The principal authors were Susana Belmartino, Carlos Bloch, Beatriz Cuenya, Jorge Hardoy, and Hilda Herzer. Dr M. Carballo and Dr A. Marin-Lira of WHO's Maternal and Child Health unit contributed additional technical material, and Mr David Satterthwaite and Ms Kate Sebag of the Human Settlements Programme, International Institute for Environment and Development, London, undertook the overall editing.

Introduction

In recent decades, most Third World countries have experienced an unprecedented growth in their urban populations. Yet little or nothing has been done to provide the homes and neighbourhoods where these growing populations live with the services and amenities essential for a healthy, adequate life: piped water, facilities for the removal of household and human wastes, storm- and surface-water drainage, all-weather access roads, and the health care and emergency life-saving services that should complement them. In virtually all countries, local and city authorities lack the power, resources, and trained personnel to meet their responsibilities in providing such services and facilities. And most countries have relatively poor economies (in terms of per capita gross domestic product) and limited natural resources. This publication will concentrate on the implications of this situation for child health. Chapter 1 reviews living conditions and health problems with special reference to child health, while Chapter 2 considers the ways in which people in lower-income groups find somewhere to live in the urban centres of the Third World. Chapter 3 discusses the role of neighbourhood organizations set up by the residents of low-income areas in tackling health problems, while Chapter 4 reviews the role of city and municipal authorities. Chapter 5 contains recommendations on the most urgently needed action by national and local governments and international agencies to deal with problems of child health in urban areas. It suggests that, in many urban neighbourhoods, collaboration between neighbourhood associations and local authorities, supported by national governments and international agencies, offers the most promising strategy for improving infant, child, and adult health.

Despite the fact that there are some common factors of great relevance to child health and survival in the scale and form of urban change in most developing countries, great care must be taken not to make sweeping generalizations. Urbanization has taken many forms in different countries or regions and at different times in history — for it reflects the society's economy, structure, and culture. It also reflects history: in most developing countries, the location of urban centres, their relative importance, and the form and layout of their central districts owe much to developments under colonial rule while, in many of them, precolonial influences are also evident. Thus, few valid generalizations can be made about urbanization in the Third World; there are very large variations in the proportions of national populations living in urban centres and their distribution in centres of different sizes. Each country has its own unique and complex mix of economic, social, political, ecological, and demographic characteristics which influence the form that urbanization takes. Thus, this publication will concentrate on the action needed to improve child health in growing urban centres where the local authorities — whatever form they take — lack the investment capacity needed to offer an entire city population the standard of services and facilities essential to health, generally found in the developed countries.

The gap between needs and responses

Although precise data on the spatial distribution of urban populations are limited (as are analyses of the relationship between this distribution and socioeconomic factors), it is clear that urbanization is now assuming features that are very different from those of the past and have different implications for the populations concerned. Over the past century, there has been an unprecedented increase both in total urban population and in the proportion of the total population living and working in urban centres. It is also evident that very few national governments or international agencies have been able to respond adequately to the housing and health problems that have accompanied this change. While a number of interventions to deal with such problems have been considered or applied, these have tended to be on a very small scale in relation to the need. In addition, they have almost always been sectoral — for instance, the construction of "low-cost" housing units. However, a multisectoral approach is needed, since the problems in question arise from a combination of inadequate incomes and of housing, living, and working environments that expose people to numerous diseases, infections, and chemical and physical hazards. Improving the health of infants, children, young people, and adults demands action not only by health agencies but by those working in the areas of housing, planning, public works, transport, pollution control, and education.

Thus, the poverty that is so often associated with urbanization, especially in developing countries in recent decades, has remained relatively untouched, while the scale of the problem it presents continues to grow. The rapid growth of cities has usually been associated with a rapid increase in the number of people living in overcrowded accommodation, much of it built illegally, with little or no provision for piped water, sanitation, collection and disposal of household waste, or health care. In addition, for substantial proportions of most cities' populations, incomes are both inadequate and unstable.

To date, attempts by governments and international agencies to address such problems have been concentrated in the larger cities or metropolitan areas. Considerable attention has been focused on cities such as São Paulo, Brazil, the population of which, according to United Nations projections, will increase to 24 million by the year 2000, or Calcutta, India (projected population, 16.6 million), or the metropolitan area of Mexico City (projected population, 26 million) (*90a*). Concern for cities such as these, for which the demographic projections may be somewhat exaggerated, has tended to draw attention away from small and intermediate-size urban centres. In many countries, these contain more than half the total urban population and many are, in fact, growing faster than the larger urban centres. Their poorer inhabitants are usually facing problems comparable in scale and kind to those of poorer groups in larger metropolitan centres as regards inability to obtain adequate incomes and access to basic services and facilities (*37*). The deterioration of the human habitat may be a much more widespread phenomenon than has hitherto been realized, affecting not only large cities but many smaller urban centres whose populations are also growing at a rate with which the provision of social and environmental services cannot keep up.

The question remains whether the change in emphasis evident on the part of some governments and aid agencies towards more support for smaller urban centres responds to predetermined priorities that may be based on inadequate analyses, or whether it reflects the conclusion that the large agglomerations have now become unmanageable and that attention should be focused on those smaller cities where national and international resources may make a greater impact. If the latter is the case, there remains the question of what is likely to happen to the larger metropolitan areas, which would, with this rationalization of resources, be relatively neglected. Many smaller urban centres may have grown explosively in the last few decades, as is the case with the national capitals in most sub-Saharan African nations — the population of Nouakchott, Mauritania, for example, increased from 5800 in 1965 to 250 000 in 1982 (*87*) — and certain small or intermediate urban centres in more urbanized nations like Machala, Ecuador, whose population expanded from 7549 to 105 521 between 1950 and 1982 (*49*).

Where one or two very large metropolitan centres have developed within a country, their growth rates have often slowed down considerably in recent years, but because these rates are calculated on such a large base population, these centres can still account for a high proportion of total urban population growth. For example, population growth in Mexico City and Lima in recent years has, in each case, been several times that of the country's 8–10 next largest cities. While natural population increase is the chief factor in their growth, such cities may also remain major foci of rural–urban migration. The lack of explicit answers to the questions thus raised, reflects the general absence of any national policy — or policy on the part of international agencies — with regard to urbanization and the amelioration or improvement of the quality of life associated with rapid urban growth.

Although national development plans often state an interest in improving the physical and social environment of low-income urban groups, few countries have actually initiated systematic improvement programmes on a scale likely to have an impact. Neither national nor city authorities have extended basic services, such as piped water and the organized collection and disposal of household wastes, or basic infrastructure (e.g., electricity, roads, and storm drainage) to the already underprovided lower-income urban population. They have also proved unable to guarantee the needed supply of new residential land-plots at prices that would allow lower-income (or indeed middle-income) groups to organize the construction of their own houses. The inevitable result has been a rapid growth in the number of people inadequately housed — for instance, in overcrowded, deteriorating tenement buildings or in squatter settlements and other forms of illegal residential development. Many cities also contain tens of thousands of people who literally have no accommodation at all and sleep on pavements, in parks or other open spaces, or in recesses of public buildings.

This is not just a problem in the poorer Third World countries, most of which had very small urban populations in 1950 and little in the way of the legal and institutional structures needed to address urban problems. It is also evident in most of the richer Third World countries, including those where rapid urbanization began in the late nineteenth and early twentieth centuries. Even in those where there have been major building programmes (and where the number of conventional dwellings constructed per 1000 inhabitants during the 1960s and 1970s was highest, e.g., Argentina, Brazil, Chile, Cuba, Malaysia, Mexico, the Republic of Korea, Thailand, Tunisia, and Uruguay), total output was far below the growth in population or in number of households, and was certainly insufficient to replace substandard units and lessen overcrowding. In most of these countries, the bulk of the new housing was in the larger urban agglomerations and not in the intermediate or smaller cities.

The lack of resources

Multilateral and bilateral aid programmes have reflected the low priority given by national governments to their mounting housing problems and backlogs in the provision of basic services and facilities; between 1980 and 1984, just 1.6% of aid went to housing and urban and community development, with just 3.5% to water, sanitation, and drainage.[1] Multilateral aid in these areas tended to concentrate on the largest cities. Claiming that they reflect the priorities set by national governments, major international agencies, such as the World Bank, have focused aid on the larger urban centres. In Latin America, 60.6% of the loans approved by the World Bank for work on housing, urban transport, water supply, sewage, and building materials, during the period 1970–79, and 49.3% of the loans made by the Inter-American Development Bank between 1970 and 1978 went to projects in national capitals and, as a second priority, to cities with populations over 500 000 (12). There was a comparable concentration of such aid in national capitals and large cities in other regions. Of the 11 cities that have received most multilateral aid for shelter-related projects during the period 1980–84 (in excess of US$ 80 million in each case), seven were national capitals, and all but one of the rest were metropolitan areas with populations of over 2 million. But even these, the cities most favoured by multilateral aid, received far less than was needed; a recent evaluation of the needs of São Paulo suggested that US$ 50 billion would be required over the next 15 years in order simply to maintain the present, already inadequate, standards.

To date, there is no indication as to where capital investment on the scale required can be obtained. The combination of inadequate investment in urban development, often a result of poorly defined priorities, and the low priority given by multilateral and bilateral agencies to improving the housing and living conditions of lower-income groups and their access to basic services raises the crucial question of how, during a period of significant economic recession, governments in countries that are heavily in debt can cope with the administrative and managerial problems of urbanization.

Almost 50% of today's Third World population is estimated to live in conditions of extreme poverty (28). The severely detrimental social, psychological, and physical effects of this on children, especially in an urban setting, have seldom been recognized. Poor housing, inadequate and often contaminated water supply, overcrowding,

---

[1] UNITED NATIONS CENTRE FOR HUMAN SETTLEMENTS (HABITAT). *Finance and other assistance provided to and among developing countries for human settlements*: report of the Executive Director. Nairobi, 1986 (document HS/C/9/6).

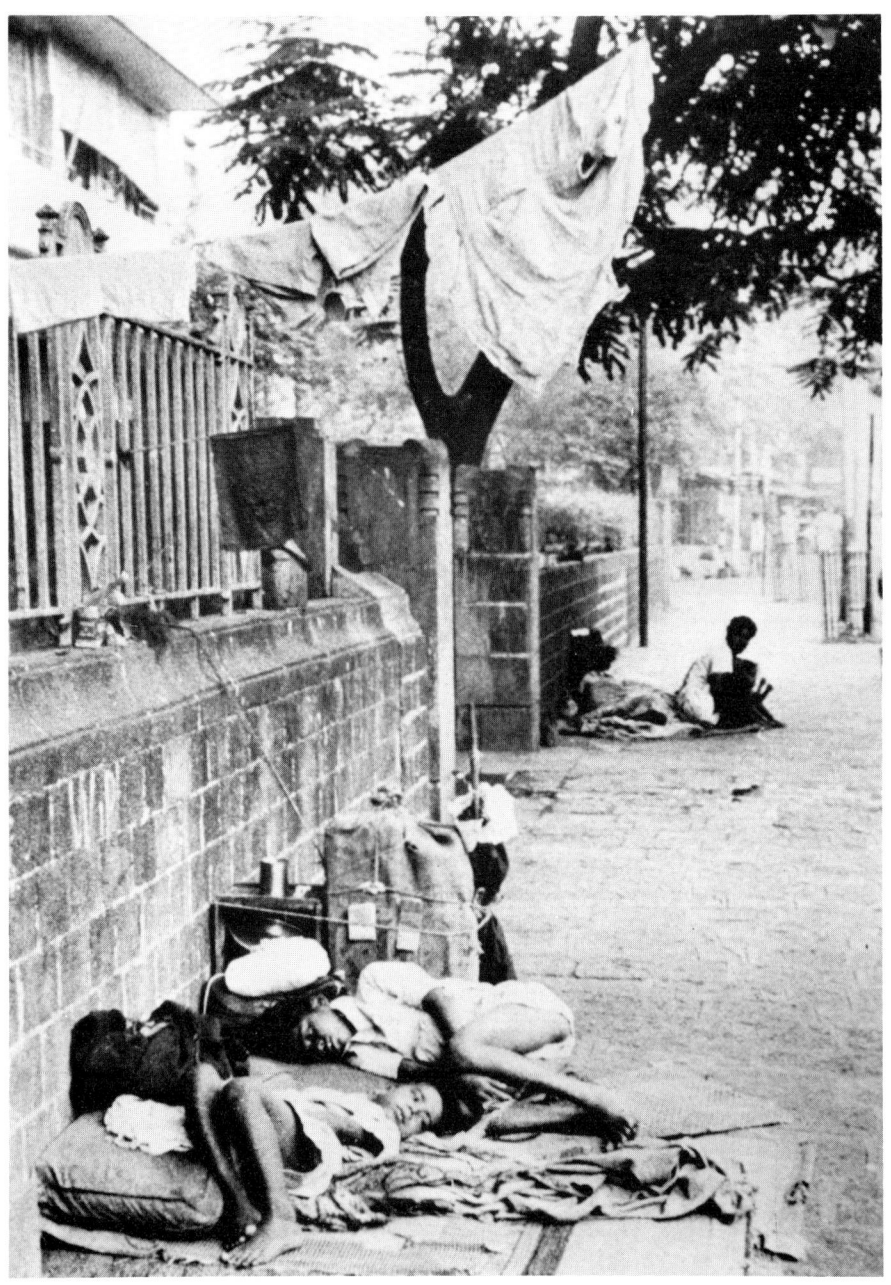

Photo WHO/UNICEF/J. Ling

Some 100 million people in the world have no housing at all.

poor waste disposal, and poor sanitation quickly translate into malnutrition, respiratory infections, diarrhoeal diseases and other waterborne infections, accidents, and retarded growth. These are largely products of the urban environment. Lack of parental supervision, child abandonment, early childhood labour, and other social problems associated with poverty proliferate within the poorer areas of cities.[1]

The fact that more children were born in the period 1960–1980 than in the two preceding decades and that increasing proportions of children are born and grow up in urban environments makes the problem of urbanization and its impact on child health all the more critical. Although the chances of child survival may in aggregate have improved, children's chances of living a sound, healthy life have not. For a large number of infants and children, the future in the context of contemporary urban growth is very bleak. In many squatter settlements where there is no safe water supply for the inhabitants or facilities for the removal of household and human wastes, a child born today is 40–50 times more likely to die before the age of 5 years than one born at the same moment in a prosperous developed country. The future is also bleak, even for Third World governments intent on improving conditions, because of mounting debt problems, frequent economic stagnation, and a shortage of trained personnel.

The national and international resources devoted to the social, psychological, and physical health needs of children living in urban tenements, squatter settlements, and other inadequate environments have been even more limited than those devoted to the wider categories of housing and improvement of the physical environment. In addition, many "low-income" housing programmes have never reached the lower-income groups for whom they were intended while others have had the net effect of further impoverishing the communities involved, precisely because they failed to understand or give due attention to the social and health dimensions of poverty.

Thus the task facing governments and international agencies is to slow down, halt, and then reverse the current trend of a progressive increase in the numbers of infants and children dying, being permanently disabled, or being repeatedly sick or injured from accidents and diseases that are easily prevented through the provision of basic services, facilities, and support for improved housing and

---

[1] ROSSI-ESPAGNET, A. *Primary health care in urban areas; reaching the urban poor in developing countries. A state-of-the-art report.* Unpublished UNICEF/WHO document, SHS 84.4.

living conditions. During the last two decades, research in low-income settlements and work with community organizations have laid the foundation for a better understanding of the relationship between the physical environment and poverty, and their impact on health and community conditions (4, 11, 24, 39, 59, 88, 94)[1,2] as well as on the physical health of communities (9, 41).[3]

---

[1] ROSSI-ESPAGNET, A. *Primary health care in urban areas: reaching the urban poor in developing countries. A state-of-the-art report.* Unpublished UNICEF/WHO document, SHS 84.4.

[2] WORLD HEALTH ORGANIZATION. *Shelter and health* (contribution of the World Health Organization to the International Year of Shelter for the Homeless). Unpublished WHO document, EHE/RUD/87.1.

[3] MASON, S. P. & STEPHENS, B. *Housing and health: an analysis for use in the planning, design and evaluation of low-income housing programs.* Study prepared for the Office of Housing, USAID, Washington, DC, 1981.

1
Living conditions and health problems in urban centres

Background—the global picture

The rapid growth of densely populated, predominantly low-income settlements in the cities of the Third World has come to constitute one of the most serious threats to health. Available statistical information and studies based on evaluations of living conditions in low-income settlements (20), suggest that three major types of pathology are emerging:

(a) infectious and gastrointestinal diseases, often termed "diseases of poverty" (these have, by and large, disappeared from developed countries, but are today a major source of morbidity and mortality in children in the developing world);

(b) chronic degenerative diseases associated with poor living and working conditions;

(c) pathogenic conditions associated with stress often precipitated by social isolation, insecurity, dissolution of primary (family) relations, and cultural conflict where there is rapid urban development.

With regard to infectious and gastrointestinal diseases, it is currently estimated that up to 44.4% of all deaths in children under 4 years of age can be directly accounted for by repeated episodes of diarrhoeal disease.[1] Fourteen surveys in the African Region of WHO and 17 in its Eastern Mediterranean Region gave similarly high rates.[1] Children affected by serious diarrhoeal diseases in these countries are likely to spend up to 20% of their first 2 years of life suffering from serious diarrhoea, with a median number of 4.9 episodes per child per year (83). Respiratory infections and nutritional deficiencies, both of which are closely associated with poverty, overcrowding, and poor environmental conditions,

---

[1] *Diarrhoeal Diseases Control Programme: fourth programme report, 1983–1984.* Unpublished WHO document, WHO/CDD/85.13.

constitute the two other major causes of morbidity and mortality in young children (Fig. 1 and Fig. 2).

Infant mortality rates, computed for the major geographical regions, are improving overall, but are still high in Africa where the estimated average rate for 1980–85 was 116 per 1000 live births.[1] South Asia and Latin America follow closely with rates estimated at over 100 and 63, respectively, per 1000 live births.[1] These are the very regions that are currently experiencing rapid urbanization resulting in the development of numerous and often large illegal settlements and ever greater numbers of tenements or cheap boarding-houses where poor environmental hygiene and physical and social conditions in general are particularly conducive to disease. The estimated number of children under 15 and under 5 years of age were 1632 million and 572 million, respectively, in 1985[2] (Fig. 3). Of these, 517 million live in urban agglomerations.

In Third World countries, approximately 31.7% of all children under 15 years of age live in urban areas, and 50% of these are considered to be living in conditions of extreme poverty — a total of 218 million in 1985 (77 million less than 5 years old). Conservative estimates suggest that, by the year 2000, poor urban children under the age of 15 years will number 253 million, with 91 million of them less than 5 years old. Given the historical patterns of natural growth among urban poor populations, the actual numbers may be considerably higher (70).[3] In addition, economic stagnation may increase the proportion of children living below the poverty line between now and the year 2000, although economic stagnation is also likely to slow down rural-to-urban migration in many countries and thus reduce the growth in urban population. The actual distribution of such children varies from one country to another. Data gathered during the 1970s and 1980s suggest that, in developing countries, the proportion of the national population living in deprived conditions in urban areas can range from 15% to 80% (Table 1). A lack of data in most countries and cities and a lack of agreed criteria as to what constitutes "deprived conditions" makes any estimate open to question. But an increasing number of studies suggest that between 30% and 60% of the population of most Third World urban centres are continuously exposed to diseases or other forms of health risk that would be removed, or enormously reduced, if the inhabitants

---

[1] UNITED NATIONS POPULATION DIVISION. Population Bulletin No. 14, New York, 1983 (document ST/ESA/SER.N/14).
[2] UNITED NATIONS POPULATION DIVISION. *World population prospects, estimates and projections as assessed in 1982.* New York, 1985 (Population Studies No. 86; document ST/ESA/SER.A/86).
[3] SAFILIOS-ROTHSCHILD, C. *Children and adolescents in slums and shanty towns in developing countries.* New York, United Nations Children's Fund (document 1277, Add.1).

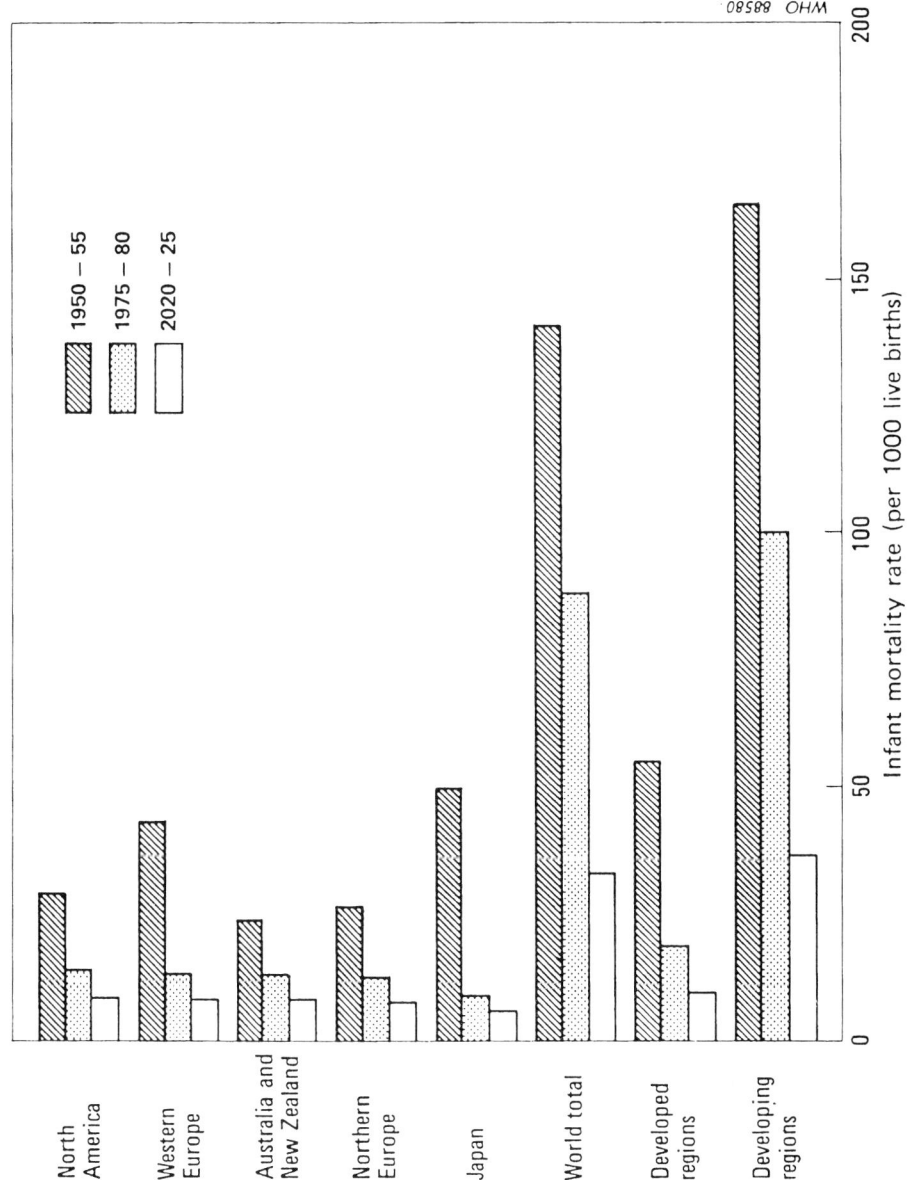

Fig. 1. Estimates and projections of infant mortality rates for 1950–55, 1975–80, and 2020–25, selected regions.
Source: Population Bulletin No. 14. New York, United Nations, 1983 (document ST/ESA/SER.N/14).

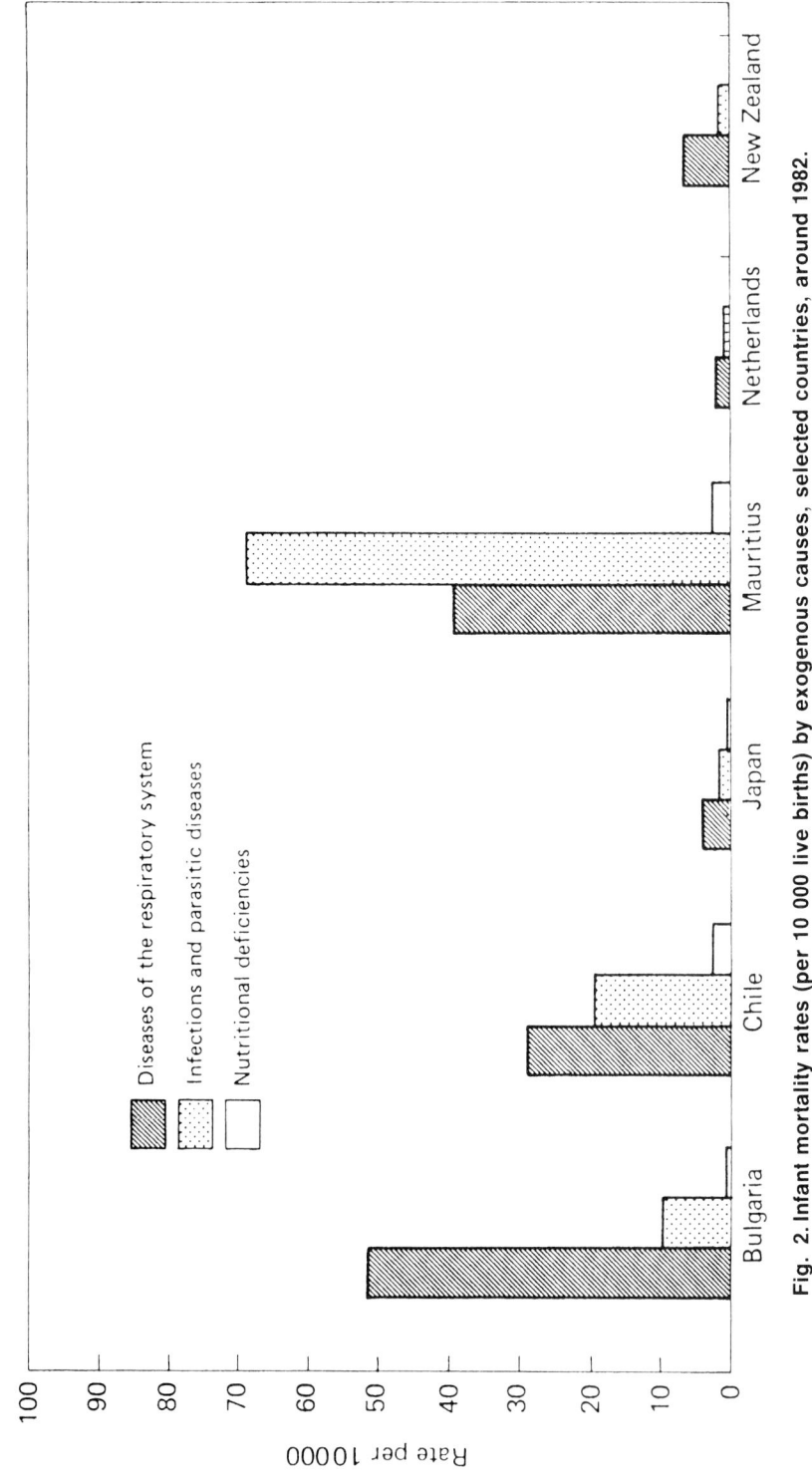

Fig. 2. Infant mortality rates (per 10 000 live births) by exogenous causes, selected countries, around 1982.

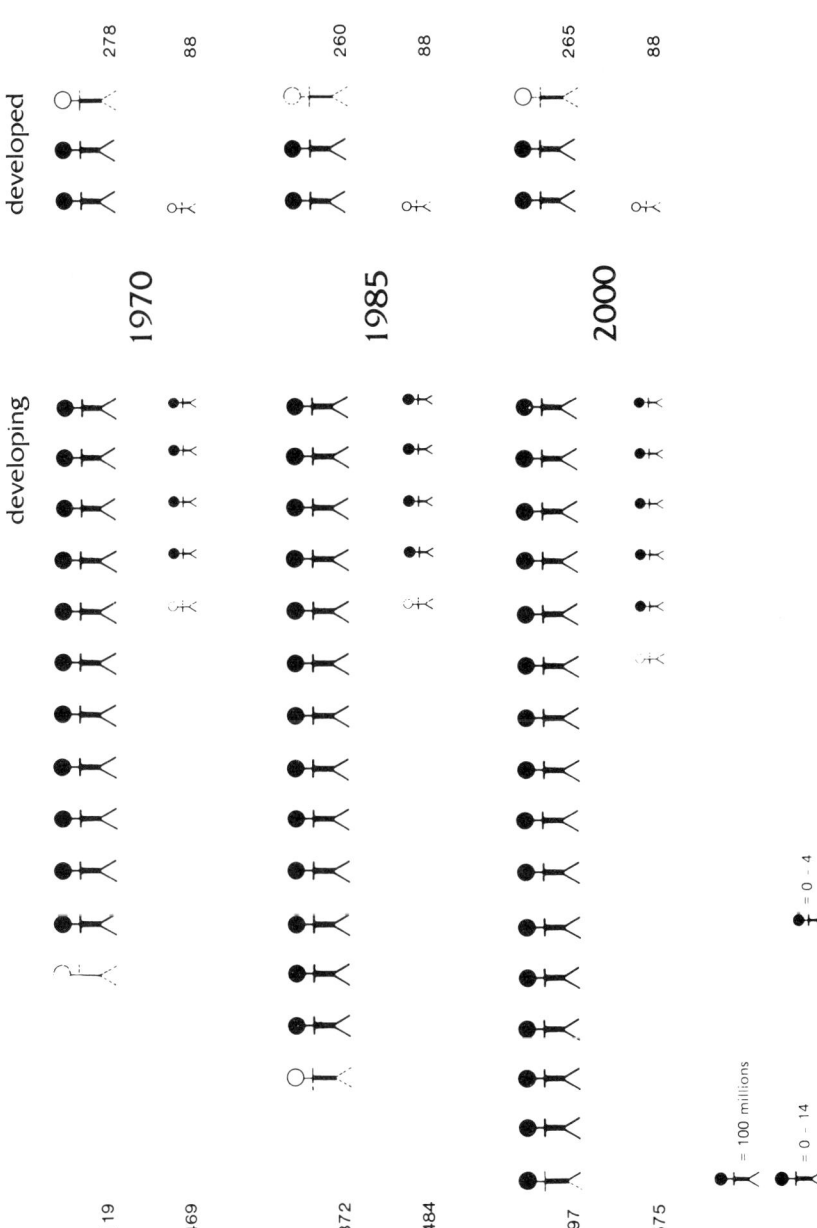

Fig. 3. Population estimates and projections for children aged 0–4 and 0–14 years in developed and developing countries, 1970, 1985, and 2000.

Table 1. Percentage of urban poor in substandard housing with inadequate or no services, 1980[a]

Country (city)	Percentage (%)	Country (city)	Percentage (%)
African Region		Chile (Santiago)	25
Angola	44–60	Colombia	54
Benin	30	Colombia (Medellín)	33[b]
Burkina Faso	62	Ecuador	53
Burundi	60	Ecuador (Guayaquil)	60–75
Cape Verde	18	El Salvador	29
Côte d'Ivoire (Abidjan)	27	Haiti (Port-au-Prince)	50
Ethiopia (Addis Ababa)	79	Mexico (Mexico City)	30–40
Gambia	20	Panama (Panama City)	73
Kenya (Nairobi)	40	Peru	33
Lesotho	59	Peru (Lima)	40
Madagascar	27	Venezuela	47
Malawi	80	**South-East Asian Region**	
Mauritania (Nouakchott)	60–70	Bangladesh	60
Mozambique (Maputo)	80	India (Bombay)	35
Niger	51	India (Calcutta)	37
Rwanda	61	India (Delhi)	56
Senegal (Dakar)	50	India (Hyderabad)	23
Sierra Leone	80	Indonesia (Jakarta)	20[c]
Somalia (Mogadiscio)	60–80	Nepal	28–31
Togo	40	Sri Lanka	42–54
European Region		Sri Lanka (Colombo)	57[d]
Turkey	25	Thailand (Bangkok)	20
Eastern Mediterranean Region		**Western Pacific Region**	
Egypt	19	Republic of Korea	5
Jordan (Amman; Zarqa)	25	Republic of Korea (Seoul)	6
Yemen	75	Fiji	10
Democratic Yemen	40	Macao	1
Region of the Americas		Malaysia (Kuala Lumpur)	25
Brazil (Porto Alegre)	15	Philippines	30
Brazil (São Paulo)	55	Solomon Islands	9
Chile	14		

[a] Based on data taken mainly from:
The International Drinking-Water Supply and Sanitation Decade. Review of national baseline data (as at 31 December 1980). Geneva, World Health Organization, 1984 (WHO Offset Publication No. 85); and *Joint UNICEF/WHO programme on equitable primary health care for urban populations: preliminary compilation of information.* Unpublished WHO document, SHS/HSR/84.1.
 The first of these sources gives data on "urban poor" for whole countries, the percentages representing total urban poor as a proportion of total urban population for each country. Data from the second source and from other sources (not listed) include "slum dwellers and squatters", or other population categories defined as having seriously substandard living conditions. The percentages quoted must therefore be interpreted with caution since the criteria by which they were calculated or estimated differ considerably. Nevertheless, the data are the best available, and demonstrate the scale and extent of the problem of inadequate accommodation.
[b] Low-income population living in 17 *barrios* or settlements.
[c] Data for 1975.
[d] Percentage of the city's total population, 1975.

had a minimal standard of secure, affordable housing with basic services and facilities. Studies of infant and child health in poor urban neighbourhoods suggest that major reductions in mortality and morbidity rates could be made by improving housing and basic services.

Water and sanitation

On the basis of information available to WHO,[1] it is estimated that, in the Third World, excluding China (for which no information was provided), at the end of 1985 only 1425 million of the total population of 2485 million had access to a water supply that was reasonably adequate and could be considered as safe, while only around 770 million had access to an appropriate form of sanitation. These figures do not even present the complete picture, since a great disparity exists between services in the urban areas and those in the rural areas, i.e., 77% of the urban population is served by water, as compared with 47% of the rural inhabitants, the corresponding figures for sanitation being 60% and 16%, respectively. However, to obtain an accurate idea of the situation, the data must be examined for regions and countries, since there are such considerable inter-regional and international disparities and global and regional estimates will be strongly influenced by conditions in the more populous countries. Suffice it to say here that, for urban water supply, coverage ranges from an estimated 62% in Africa to 90% in Central and South America, while in rural areas the range is from 31% in Africa to 62% in the Western Pacific; in the case of sanitation, the urban average ranges from 32% in South-East Asia to 88% in the Western Pacific, while the rural average is at the very low level of 7% in South-East Asia, rising to a reputed 58% in the Western Pacific. It is worth noting that the situation in the least developed countries is generally worse than in other developing countries.

Even these figures may belie the true situation, since the existence of sewerage systems in cities does not necessarily imply the proper treatment of waste. The direct outflow of sewage into rivers is common and, given the tendency to use river water as a source of drinking-water, the problem of infection is, in some cases, exacerbated. A WHO survey in selected developing countries (*56*) suggested that 1000 million people did not have any access to uncontaminated water.

---

[1] WORLD HEALTH ORGANIZATION. *International Drinking Water Supply and Sanitation Decade: mid-decade progress review.* Unpublished WHO document, A/39/11.

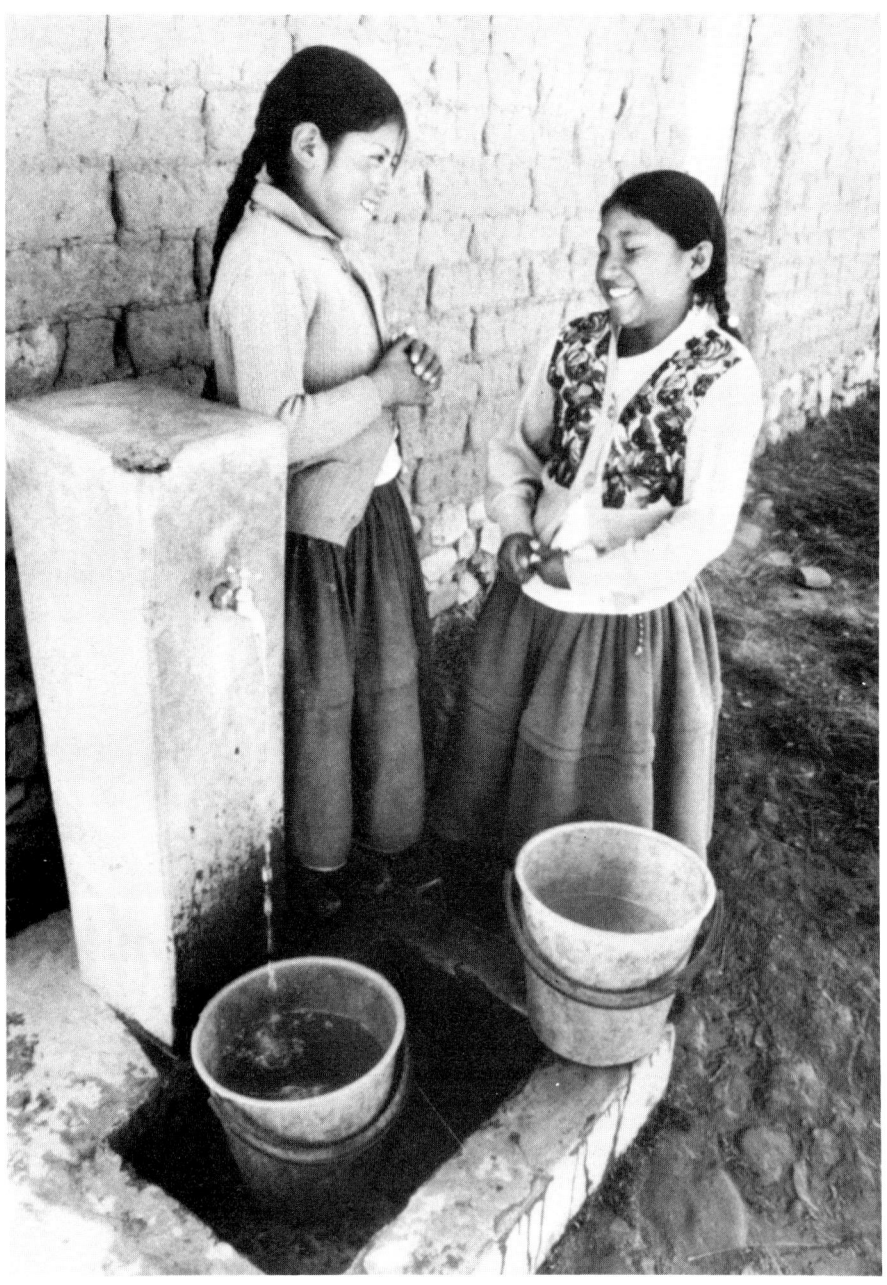

Photo WHO/PAHO/D. Downie

Safe water on tap—an essential element of primary health care.

In addition, people supplied with "piped water" from a communal tap 100 m from the house they live in (and thus in the category of "having piped water supply") are unable to use as much water as those with a supply piped directly into the house. The quantity of water available to a household has an important influence on health; no household is likely to make a liberal use of water to wash clothes or cooking and eating utensils, or for personal hygiene, if it has to be carried a long distance with the possibility of long queues at the tap. Piped water supplies are often contaminated by sewage seeping into the network when water pressure drops in an overloaded and poorly maintained distribution system. The existence of sewers does not guarantee the hygienic removal of faecal matter; sewers often run into the rivers or lakes from which many people in low-income groups draw their water.

Air and water pollution

Rivers and lakes that are used by large numbers of city inhabitants as a source of water for drinking, washing, and cooking often receive untreated industrial waste which presents serious health hazards — as can be seen by the increasing number of deaths and disablities resulting from heavy metal poisoning in Third World cities (*33, 62, 82, 84*). Untreated liquid wastes from industries and sewers or open drains are seriously damaging riverine, estuarine, and coastal fisheries. This affects poorer groups, for whom fish are an important component of the diet.

Air pollution in urban centres is a major health hazard that affects all age groups but can be particularly harmful to young children. In 1967 and again in 1974, 87 cities in the Latin American region were considered to have serious or potentially serious air pollution problems. Of these, Caracas, Cordoba (Argentina), Havana, Mexico City, Montevideo, Santiago, and São Paulo (Brazil) were considered to be the most affected. In almost every one of the cities where air quality was measured, the monthly averages for sedimentable dust were higher than the WHO guideline of 0.50 mg/cm^2; Mexico City, for example, had averages varying between 2.11 and 3.26 mg/cm^2. For the following cities, estimates of dust in suspension gave values considerably higher than the guideline level (100 μg/m^3): Buenos Aires (167.4 μg/m^3), Mexico City (145 μg/m^3), and São Paulo (169 μg/m^3) (*72*).

Rarely do data on air or water pollution include assessments of the impact on human health, least of all child health. But in the hundreds of Third World urban centres with high concentrations of heavy industries, this impact can be very significant. For instance, in 1980 in the industrial city of Cubatão, Brazil, 40 out of every 1000 babies were stillborn, while 40 others died in the first week of life, the majority of these being deformed; in a population of 80 000, over 40 000 emergency medical calls were registered, more than 10 000 being concerned with tuberculosis, pneumonia, bronchitis, emphysema, asthma, and related nose and throat ailments (*42*).

Just as the use of open fires or inefficient cooking stoves can produce indoor pollution levels capable of seriously aggravating respiratory problems, the concentration of wood and coal fires and stoves in cities can exacerbate air pollution; indeed, in many cities, these have become the major source of air pollution. City-based power stations and industries burning coal or oil with a high sulfur content often make a major contribution to air pollution. While air pollution problems created by internal combustion engines might be assumed to be relatively less serious in Third World cities where the proportion of cars to inhabitants is comparatively low, they may in fact be greater than in cities elsewhere. The combination of traffic congestion, narrow streets, lack of wind to disperse pollutants, old and poorly maintained cars, trucks, motor-cycles, and buses, plus high levels of lead additives in gasoline, often create higher concentrations of lead and carbon monoxide than are found in "western" cities. In addition, in some of the richer Asian and Latin American cities, the proportion of automobiles to inhabitants is comparable to that found in many "western" cities.

Health hazards of poverty

The scale of ill health

Recent case studies in squatter settlements have revealed a very high level of premature death and ill health, especially among infants and children. In 1984, for instance, a survey in Chheetpur, a squatter settlement with 500 inhabitants in the city of Allahabad, India, found that 55% of the children and 45% of the adults had worm infestations, while 60% had scabies. Most of the population had intakes of less than 1500 calories a day; 90% of infants and children under the age of 4 had intakes significantly below their needs. Over a period of 14 years, 143 deaths of children had been recorded. Malaria was the most commonly identified cause of death, followed by tetanus, injuries from accidents and burns, and diarrhoea, dysentery, or cholera. The site of the settlement was subject to flooding in the rainy season and lack of drainage meant that stagnant pools were present for much of the year. There were only two standpoints to meet the water needs of the entire population, and there was no public provision for sanitation or rubbish removal (*59*).

A study in Wadi Riman, a squatter settlement in Amman, Jordan, found that, per 1000 live births, 86.1 children had died before the age

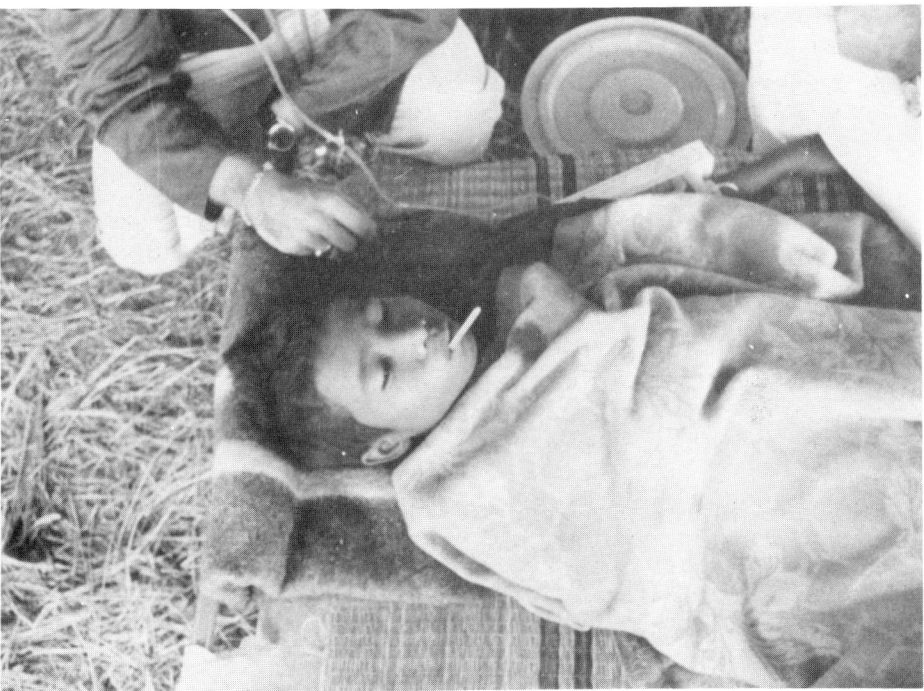

Photo WHO/M. de Vreede

A child with cerebral malaria awaits admission to hospital.

of 3, even though virtually all households had piped water and electricity and most had pit latrines. By the age of 3, nearly half of the children were infected with one or more intestinal parasites, and nearly one-third had suffered an acute respiratory infection in the period immediately preceding the survey. When the houses surveyed were divided into three groups according to the quality of construction and the materials used, the proportion of children dying before the age of 3 was significantly greater for the lower categories of house quality; in the lowest category, the rate was 109.8 per 1000 live births. The death rate for children was also significantly higher in households with less than the median income and those where mothers were illiterate rather than "probably literate" (*11*).

A study of 7 different "hutment" settlements in Poona, India, compared the health status of their inhabitants with the quality of the housing environment and the quality of the water and latrine services (*7*). The results clearly suggested a correlation between the quality of the housing/living environment and health; the incidence of ill health in children in the "best" settlements was 30–50% lower than that in the worst.

The researchers also argued that a significant proportion of the malnutrition seen among children in Poona was precipitated by disease due to the state of the physical environment.

Recent case studies suggest that health problems may be more serious for the urban poor than for rural dwellers. For instance, in the slums of Haiti's capital, Port-au-Prince, the infant mortality rate was found to be 200 per 1000 live births with another 100 per 1000 dying between their first and second birthdays; these were almost 3 times the equivalent rates in the country's rural areas (*76*). The infant mortality rate in the *bustees* of Delhi, India's capital, was found to be 221 per 1000 live births and twice as much for some of the lowest castes.[1] In Manila, the capital and by far the largest city of the Philippines, the infant mortality rate in squatter communities was found to be 3 times the average for the rest of the city; the proportion of people with tuberculosis was also 9 times higher and diarrhoea was twice as common (*9*).

It thus appears that high levels of infant and child mortality and morbidity (and indeed, high levels of ill health for all age groups) are closely associated with income (or in rural areas, access to land). In cities whose population growth has been largely the result of an influx of people from rural areas in recent decades, some of the mortality and morbidity patterns seen in low-income groups will have their origins in the rural conditions from which people have moved. Nevertheless, in the city low income, insecurity as regards housing, lack of services and facilities, and overcrowding are likely to make the most significant impact on health; the higher rate of child deaths in the Amman squatter community among households with lower than medium incomes and the especially high infant mortality rate among lower castes in Delhi are but two examples. Moreover, the health problems of members of poor households who have always lived in cities are usually much the same as those of recent migrants.

Thus, the urban poor can be regarded as the interface between underdevelopment and industrialization, and their disease pattern often reflects the problems of both. From the first they acquire a heavy burden of infectious disease and malnutrition, and from the second the wide range of chronic and social diseases that is becoming typical of urban centres in developing countries. Three main groups of health hazards have a synergistic impact on the poor. The first includes poor education, insufficient nutrition, overcrowding,

---

[1] ROSSI-ESPAGNET, A. *Primary health care in urban areas: reaching the urban poor in developing countries. A state-of-the-art report.* Unpublished UNICEF/WHO document, SHS 84.4.

and underprotection leading to excessive vulnerability and exposure to pathogenic agents, and hence to infectious diseases and malnutrition. The second relates more specifically to man-made conditions of the urban environment, including pollution, exposure to unregulated traffic, stress and alienation leading to cardiovascular, neoplastic, and mental diseases, and accidents in the home, at work, and on the road. Cardiovascular disease rates in the urban areas of developing countries for example, are often as high as those in industrialized cities, but without the corresponding resources to deal with them.[1] The third group of hazards reflects the environmental neglect that is common where national or local finances are unable to meet needs in vector control and environmental engineering. The community awareness needed to supplement the institutional contribution made by local and national governments may also be lacking (15).

Malnutrition

This is perhaps the most apparent and pervasive of the health problems of poverty resulting from the synergism mentioned above. It has been estimated (66) that the energy and protein intakes of some 145 million children under 5 years old are insufficient (Table 2).

Although malnutrition has traditionally been considered as the product of food shortage, there is growing evidence that it is a far more complex problem involving an interplay of factors of which shortage of food is only one. Inadequate preparation and storage of food, lack of knowledge about nutritional needs in infancy and childhood, and the effects of repeated infectious diseases are equally important.[2] Research on child care practices in developing countries has pointed to the importance, in this context, of the family and its role in achieving and maintaining health. Yet rapid urbanization and the associated large-scale rural-to-urban migration tend to erode the cohesive force that a family might otherwise bring to the physical and social health of its members. One reason is that the migrants are often predominantly young people, and sometimes predominantly young men or young women; this can mean highly imbalanced sex ratios and very few older people in many poorer residential neighbourhoods within cities. It often means that there are no family members available to help with child-care and child-rearing, whereas traditionally, the extended family has been important in rural areas in helping with child care and household tasks. In

---

[1] ROSSI-ESPAGNET, A. *Primary health care in urban areas: reaching the urban poor in developing countries. A state-of-the-art report.* Unpublished UNICEF/WHO document, SHS 84.4.
[2] COEYTAUX, F. *The role of the family in health: appropriate research methods.* Unpublished WHO document, FHE 84.2.

Table 2. Protein-energy malnutrition: estimated prevalence in infants under 5 years of age by region[a]

Region	Estimated prevalence[b]	
	percentage affected	number affected (millions)
Africa	25.6	21.9
Americas[c]	17.7	8.6
Asia[d]	54.0	114.6
Oceania[e]	11.5	0.3
Total	—	145.4

[a] From: *Weekly epidemiological record*, **59** (25): 190 (1984).
[b] These numbers give only a very broad estimate of trends on the basis of surveys carried out between 1973 and 1983. The prevalence is determined as the percentage of children more than 2SD below the National Child Health Standard median weight-for-age.
[c] Excluding temperate countries.
[d] Excluding USSR and North-East Asia; weighted for India.
[e] Excluding Australia and New Zealand.
Note. Traditionally, weight-for-age has been the most common indicator used in determining the prevalence of protein-energy malnutrition; it is now known that weight-for-age is a composite indicator of weight-for-height (wasting) and height-for-age (stunting).

addition, one or more members of the family may have to be highly mobile within the city (or the wider city region) to obtain income; for instance, one parent within a nuclear family may spend weeks or months away as seasonal or casual jobs become available elsewhere. In addition, the survival of poorer households often demands that both parents work with the result that infants and children have to be left in the care of others (often other children). In the lower-income groups, there is also a high proportion of households headed by women, whose role as main income-earner leaves them with little time to supervise their children (*60*).

The urban environment and the process of urbanization often involve an additional factor affecting food intake, namely — for want of a better term—"delocalization of food access". In rural areas, access to food tends to be direct and close; even though it may be in short supply, individuals or households usually have a variety of established ways of obtaining food: for example, growing it, bartering for it, collecting it, or purchasing it within a well-established price range. In the urban environment, especially in larger cities, a markedly different relationship exists between food production, food purchase, and food use. Opportunities for the home production of food are more limited, the possibility of obtaining it by barter is also limited, food markets operate in a different way, and prices are invariably higher. There are comparable differences as regards access to fuel for cooking and for heating water and the house itself. Although, in many rural areas, firewood has to be bought rather than gathered freely, it is generally more difficult and more expensive for low-income urban dwellers to obtain fuel, especially in large cities.

Not surprisingly, malnutrition has become a serious concern in many city-based, low-income communities. Average energy intake is often half to two-thirds, and vitamin A intake one-third to half of the overall city averages. Up to 50% of the children may show signs of malnutrition, 10% of them in a severe form (*9*). Observations from Abidjan (*46*), Allahabad, India (*59*), Buenos Aires (*24*), New Delhi (*26, 27*), Santiago (*3*), São Paulo, Brazil (*80*), and other cities all point to comparable patterns of malnutrition. Where it has been possible to break down the available information by socioeconomic background, it has been found that the availability of nutrients is often lower in urban populations than among corresponding rural groups (*63*) or that there are more severely malnourished children in low-income urban areas than in corresponding rural areas (*58, 93*). In a survey in India (*2*) it was reported that total morbidity among 284 children between 1 month and 5 years of age living in one urban slum area was significantly higher than it was among children living in two other areas of the same city. Upper respiratory tract infections, fever, diarrhoea, vomiting, and measles were the most frequently observed ailments in all three groups of children surveyed. Stomatitis and whooping cough were common in the urban slums.

Water-related diseases of poverty

The sheer scale and variety of the diseases related to water can be seen from Table 3, while Table 4 shows estimated reductions in morbidity as a result of improvements in water and sanitation.

A variety of diarrhoeal diseases, often exacerbating or precipitating malnutrition, account for a large part of the mortality seen in children under 2 years of age. The particularly high prevalence of these diseases in slums and shanty towns is explained by the environmental hazards typical of such areas, especially the scarcity of water, the fact that available water is often contaminated, and the lack of sewers or other means of ensuring the hygienic disposal of human wastes. Overcrowding, poor housing conditions, a high density of insects and rodents, lack of garbage disposal facilities, poor personal hygiene and/or poor hygienic conditions generally, all of which are typical of the urban slum and squatter environment, are

Table 3. Diseases related to water supply and sanitation: control measures[a]

Disease	Type and importance of control measures[b]					
	improvement in water quality	improvement in water supply quantity/convenience	personal and domestic hygiene	wastewater disposal/drainage	excreta disposal	food hygiene
Diarrhoea:						
viral diarrhoea	●	●●●	●●●	—	●●	●●
bacterial diarrhoea	●●	●●●	●●●	—	●●●	●●●
protozoal diarrhoea	●	●●●	●●●	—	●●●	●●
Poliomyelitis and hepatitis A	●	●●●	●●●	—	●●	●●
Worm infections:						
ascaris, trichuris	●	—	●	●	●●●	●
hookworm	●	●●	●●●	—	●●●	—
pinworm, dwarf tapeworm	—	●	●●●	—	●●	●●
other tapeworms	—	●	—	●	●●●	●●●
schistosomiasis	●	●●●	—	—	●●●	—
guinea-worm	●●●	—	—	—	—	—
other worms with aquatic hosts	—	—	—	—	●	—
Skin infections	—	●●●	●●●	—	—	—
Eye infections	●	●●●	●●●	●	●	—
Insect-transmitted diseases:						
malaria	—	—	—	●	—	—
urban yellow fever, dengue	—	—	●[c]	●●	—	—
bancroftian filariasis	—	—	—	●●●	●●	—
onchocerciasis	—	—	—	—	●	—

[a] From: *Intersectoral action for health*. Geneva, World Health Organization, 1986.
[b] Importance of control measures: ●●● high ●● medium ● low to negligible.
[c] Vectors breed in water storage containers.

Table 4. Potential benefits of improvements in water and sanitation[a]

Diseases	Projected reduction in morbidity (%)
Cholera, typhoid, leptospirosis, scabies, guinea-worm infection	80–100
Trachoma, conjunctivitis, yaws, schistosomiasis	60–70
Tularaemia, paratyphoid, bacillary dysentery, amoebic dysentery, gastroenteritis, louse-borne diseases, diarrhoeal disease, ascariasis, skin infections	40–50

[a] From: *Intersectoral action for health.* Geneva, World Health Organization, 1986.

predisposing factors for gastrointestinal diseases.[1] While a shortage of uncontaminated, easily available water is a problem in all developing countries, unplanned and rapid urbanization appears to be increasingly associated with the deterioration of existing water systems, whether natural or man-made. In densely populated areas where facilities for the disposal of household and industrial wastes are inadequate or non-existent, the bacterial contamination of water by industrial and human wastes is fast becoming a major problem. The close relationship between water and sanitation means that improvements in one of these areas without corresponding improvements in the other are likely to have little impact on child health. The possibility of using sewers to dispose of human wastes depends not only on the existence of pipes but on having sufficient water, while inability to dispose of human wastes endangers, in its turn, whatever water supply is available.[1]

The importance of water in transmitting disease can be seen in many areas of developing countries where what were previously primarily rural diseases, such as malaria, yellow fever, dengue, and schistosomiasis, are now becoming endemic in the cities (*95*). The transformation of schistosomiasis into an urban disease, as can be seen in São Paulo and other Brazilian cities, is also associated with the migration of individuals from rural areas of the north-east of the country, where schistosomiasis is endemic. Unplanned urbanization promoted by land speculation has, in turn, led to physical conditions

---

[1] ROSSI-ESPAGNET, A. *Primary health care in urban areas: reaching the urban poor in developing countries. A state-of-the-art report.* Unpublished UNICEF/WHO document, SHS 84.4.

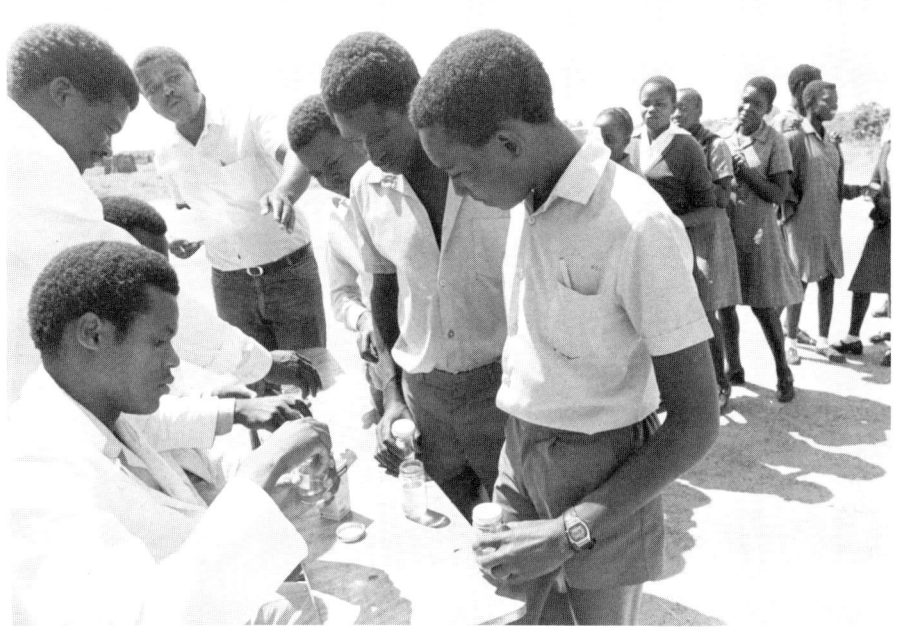

Schistosomiasis control teams are now having to work close to some of the world's sprawling cities.

that favour the transmission of the disease. Road or embankment works frequently create small lagoons on the periphery of cities, and these constitute ideal spots for the transmission of the vector (25).

The paucity of suitable facilities in urban slum and squatter settlements is often exacerbated by various kinds of social behaviour that make for poor personal hygiene and by the accumulation of stagnant water pools around homes (91, 92). In a recent survey in Chile (31), it was reported that 72% of the families studied did not boil water prior to drinking it, and 18% of them threw waste water into their backyards or other areas close to their homes; 20% of households that did not have access to regular garbage collection likewise disposed of their wastes in neighbouring vacant lots or their own backyards. But, while the promotion of behavioural changes (for example, through pamphlets and educational services) can be helpful in dealing with health problems, the changes needed (such as more careful disposal of waste water and household garbage, at some distance from the house) often demand more time and energy than are available to the members of a poor household, especially given the long hours that most of the adults have to work in order to earn what they can. It is hardly equitable to expect people in lower income groups to take responsibility for their own garbage and waste water disposal while those in middle and upper income groups are provided with sewers and services for the regular collection of their household wastes.

Respiratory diseases

A third aspect of the synergism often seen in economically disadvantaged populations, and increasingly in urban slum and squatter settlements, is the high incidence of respiratory diseases, especially among young children (Table 5). Like diarrhoeal diseases, acute respiratory infections are diseases of poverty (Table 6). Although poorly reported in most instances, respiratory diseases are thought to be the second major cause of death (with malnutrition as an underlying cause) in developing countries. A survey undertaken by the Metropolitan Development Authority in Calcutta, India's largest city, in an upgraded low-income area found that respiratory diseases were the most commonly reported of all diseases; 76.4% of the households surveyed reported that family members had suffered from respiratory diseases in the previous year, and 65.5% that they had suffered from gastrointestinal disorders (*85*). The incidence of tuberculosis was found to be 10 times that in another, "non-slum" neighbourhood nearby. In India's second largest city, Bombay, a survey by the Municipal Corporation found that tuberculosis and respiratory ailments were the main causes of death; among those living in the more polluted areas — mostly the lower income groups — much higher incidences of serious respiratory diseases were recorded (*85*).

In a study of childhood mortality carried out in Latin America (*73*), respiratory illnesses came second only to diarrhoeal infections among reported causes of death in children of less than 5 years of age (Table 7). This was the case in all 13 regions included in the study, the rates for Paraguay and Peru being 30 times higher than those reported in Canada and the USA (*68*). Overcrowding, poor ventilation, poor temperature control, and environmental pollution are all associated with respiratory infection in early childhood (*69*) and are, in turn, common to urban slum and squatter settlements and unplanned urban settlements in general.

The growth of urban areas has also generated a range of new disease-producing agents which are not necessarily related to poor environmental sanitation, namely products of chemical residues, toxic wastes, car exhaust fumes, and various synthetic products (*38, 50, 51, 54*). Recent epidemiological data (*55*) show that, in the USA, an

Table 5. Deaths from respiratory diseases in infants and children aged 1–4 years, selected developing countries[a]

Country or territory	Year	Deaths from respiratory disease				Total deaths from respiratory diseases (all ages)
		Age <1 year		Age 1–4 years		
		No.	%[b]	No.	%[b]	
Argentina	1981	2 209	16.8	542	4.1	13 123
Chile	1983	860	11.6	199	2.7	7 413
Cuba	1981	215	4.7	82	1.8	4 601
Dominican Republic	1982	432	24.8	252	14.5	1 742
El Salvador	1981	862	41.8	415	20.1	2 064
Guatemala	1981	3 618	35.5	2 366	23.2	10 185
Martinique	1982	2	2.5	0	0	80
Mauritius	1982	78	18.3	46	10.8	426
Panama	1983	116	15.7	72	9.8	738
Paraguay	1980	490	37.2	181	13.8	1 316
Peru	1981	5 211	28.1	4 126	22.3	18 535
Sri Lanka	1980	1 869	47.3	895	22.6	3 955
Venezuela	1980	1 228	25.1	602	12.3	4 891

[a] Source: *World health statistics annual, 1983, 1984, 1985.* Geneva, World Health Organization, 1983, 1984, 1985.
[b] As a percentage of all deaths due to respiratory disease.

Table 6. Deaths from pneumonia in infants and children aged 1–4 years, selected developing countries[a]

Country or territory	Year	Deaths from pneumonia				Total deaths from pneumonia (all ages)
		Age <1 year		Age 1–4 years		
		No.	%	No.	%	
Argentina	1981	1 619	26.8	381	6.3	6 038
Chile	1983	744	17.9	145	3.5	4 144
Cuba	1981	210	5.4	63	1.6	3 871
Dominican Republic	1982	252	35.8	153	21.8	703
El Salvador	1981	262	36.0	133	18.3	728
Guatemala	1981	2 115	35.3	1 540	25.7	5 984
Martinique	1982	1	5.3	0	0	19
Mauritius	1982	48	14.8	23	7.1	324
Panama	1983	61	20.5	31	10.4	297
Paraguay	1980	389	46.5	127	15.2	837
Peru	1981	3 376	26.5	2 556	20.1	12 729
Sri Lanka	1980	1 040	34.3	560	18.5	3 030
Venezuela	1980	910	31.2	440	15.1	2 917

[a] Source: *World health statistics annual, 1983, 1984, 1985.* Geneva, World Health Organization, 1983, 1984, 1985.

Table 7. Proportion of deaths of children under 5 years of age in selected Latin American countries (not due to congenital anomalies or perinatal causes), in which faeces-related disease, airborne disease, or malnutrition was the primary cause[a]

Area	Faeces-related diseases (%)	Airborne diseases (%)	Nutritional deficiency (%)	Total (%)
Argentina				
Chaco, rural	40	36	2	79
San Juan, rural	35	42	8	84
San Juan, suburban	34	38	8	80
San Juan, central urban	38	32	3	72
Bolivia				
Chaco Resistencia, rural	52	27	6	84
Viacha, rural	25	65	0	91
La Paz, urban	29	55	3	87
Brazil				
Ribeirão Prêto, rural	50	29	3	81
Ribeirão Prêto Franca, rural	55	20	7	82
Recife, urban	42	41	5	88
Ribeirão, Prêto, urban	49	36	2	87
São Paulo, urban	40	33	5	78
Chile				
Santiago, suburban	33	38	3	74
Santiago, urban	31	37	6	73
Colombia				
Cali, urban	44	25	15	84
Cartagena, urban	38	23	17	78
Medellín, urban	49	22	11	82
San Salvador				
El Salvador, rural	51	22	13	86
El Salvador, urban	52	28	6	86
Jamaica				
St. Andrew, rural	23	23	23	69
Kingston, urban	37	21	5	63

[a] Source: PUFFER, R. R. & SERRANO, C. V. *Inter-American investigation of mortality in childhood.* Provisional report. Washington, DC, Pan American Health Organization, 1971.

estimated 4% of children between 4 months and 5 years of age have blood concentrations of lead greater than 300 µg/litre, which puts them at increased risk of subtle, but persistent, cognitive and neurobehavioural deficits (74, 78). Exposure to lead from the interiors and exteriors of old and deteriorating houses has become a major cause of lead poisoning among children of preschool age (21). In low-income communities where building maintenance is poor and old materials tend to be used and reused, lead-based paint on exposed surfaces is particularly dangerous. However, airborne lead from industrial emissions or motor vehicle exhausts may have an even greater impact on health. A recent survey of 693 children living near a lead-smelting plant in Brazil (18) revealed high levels of zinc protoporphyrin (ZPP) and lead in their blood. The survey found a strong statistical association between ZPP levels and proximity to the plant, length of residence, and age. Children living in low-income areas are also likely to be living closer than others to industrial plants and thus to be exposed to a higher level of lead in the environment. Infants and women appear to be especially vulnerable to lead poisoning. Very high levels of airborne lead have been found alongside busy roads in Kuala Lumpur[1] and Zimbabwe (*1*), and also in Delhi (*84*). In children, the central nervous system is highly vulnerable and readily damaged by environmental exposure to lead, even in low doses (*64*). Additional research has suggested that children who have been chronically exposed to lead in the environment may become hyperactive, lack fine motor coordination, have a lower IQ, and experience perceptual problems (*6*). Chromosomal abnormalities have also been associated with lead poisoning.

The physical and social environment

In addition to the many infectious, chronic, and degenerative diseases associated with low-income areas in contemporary cities, the typical physical and social environment of these areas is conducive to a high incidence of domestic and street accidents (*48*). Badly planned and overcrowded houses, cheap building materials (frequently including materials from city rubbish dumps), and the use of open fires or unguarded stoves increase the risk of young children being harmed by falls, burns, and accidental poisoning. The impact of accidental injuries on health is greatly increased by the fact that there are rarely facilities for first aid, for emergency life-saving, or even for ensuring hospital treatment at all. The association of a low level of literacy among adults and the physical and social environment of urban slum and squatter settlements has tended to make programmes of preventive action difficult, especially in families that are, for economic reasons, constantly on the move to different parts of the city.

Although less well described and poorly documented, psychosocial problems have been reported among children and adolescents living in low-income urban areas. The urban environment, particularly when characterized by poverty, overcrowding, poor environmental sanitation, and lack of space for children's play and recreation, can be particularly detrimental to those in the younger age groups. As indicated earlier, the rapid rural–urban migration that has contributed significantly to total population growth in many cities

---

[1] SANI, S. *Urbanization and the atmospheric environment in Southeast Asia.* Paper presented at the Seminar of Development, Environment, and the Natural Resource Crisis in Asia and the Pacific, Penang, Malaysia, October 1983.

in recent decades may be sex- and age-selective. For instance, rural households often support the move of one adult member to an urban centre in search of employment, while one or more adult members may seek temporary urban employment at times when there is little work in rural areas. The migration patterns that have become an integral part of the strategy for survival of so many households may undermine extended family and kinship systems that had previously provided continuity and security for young children (52). The cultural conflict often associated with migration from traditional rural communities to large metropolitan areas creates a degree of insecurity in the family that permeates all age groups and quickly begins to affect the youngest members. Many of the physical ailments in young children, including chronic diseases, may to some extent be due to a lack of emotional security and an absence of appropriate rearing practices providing for a continuity of caregivers (54).

2
Housing and health

Background

A key factor in the rapid growth of shanty towns and slum districts in the Third World has been the emergence of large urban populations characterized by considerable inequalities in income. A high proportion of these city-dwellers have little or no possibility of buying or renting a house with basic services, or even of buying a legitimate plot, with connections for water and sewers, on which a house can be built. Even the cheapest house or apartment with minimum services is too expensive for them.

All city-dwellers need to have access to affordable accommodation offering adequate space, a ready and sufficient supply of potable water and electricity, and provision for the hygienic disposal of human wastes. They also need housing sites and neighbourhoods with provision for surface-water drainage and for the removal of household wastes. Children need space for play, sport, and recreation that is free from obvious health hazards—for instance, without any stagnant pools contaminated with faecal matter, hazardous chemical agents, or household garbage. Similarly, measures are needed to keep such areas free from road traffic. Sufficient living space is also important, given the high incidence of accidents to children in the home; cramped and overcrowded houses often make it difficult or impossible to safeguard children against the hazards presented by open fires or stoves or by chemicals and medicines kept in the house. The nine features of the housing environment listed below have important direct or indirect effects on health; in each instance, the health problems created by these factors can be eliminated, or much reduced, by appropriate public and community action (*97*).

Factors in the housing environment with an effect on health

1. **The house as a structure and shelter.** Makeshift dwellings do not provide protection against extremes of heat and cold; they lack insulation against noise and invasion by dust, rain, insects,

and rodents. Chagas' disease, which affects 16 to 18 million people in Latin America, is transmitted by bugs that live and breed in cracks in the walls of mud or wooden houses. In the case of small, cramped dwellings made of temporary materials and containing open fires or unprotected stoves, the risk of accidental fires, burns and scalds is high.

2. **Water and drinking-water supplies.** Water is a primary medium for the transmission of diseases, the most important of which are typhoid, cholera, hepatitis, poliomyelitis, dysentery, amoebiasis, and infection by intestinal protozoa.

3. **Excreta, sewage, and solid waste disposal.** Human excreta are among the most dangerous substances with which people can come into contact; they are the principal source of the pathogenic organisms of many communicable diseases, particularly infections of the intestinal tract (enteric diseases). There is a direct link between absence of facilities for the safe disposal of excreta and solid wastes and the incidence of infections due to the contamination of food, water, or the fingers by faecal matter containing pathogenic organisms and the subsequent ingestion of these organisms by susceptible individuals. Pathogens include certain bacteria and viruses, and intestinal parasites (hookworm, ascaris, whipworm, pinworm, threadworm).

4. **Land.** Housing sites and nearby open space contaminated with faecal matter, chemicals, and other wastes pose major health risks, especially for children playing on them. Many settlements have been developed on land subject to flooding or landslides. Poor site drainage can result in waterlogged soil, which is an ideal medium for the transmission of parasitic diseases, such as hookworm. Pools of standing water may become contaminated and transmit enteric diseases; they also serve as ideal breeding-grounds for mosquito pests and vectors, thus contributing to the spread of filariasis, malaria, and other diseases.

5. **Overcrowding.** Small, poorly ventilated dwellings promote the spread of communicable diseases by aerosol droplets: for instance, influenza, tuberculosis, meningitis, all of which are associated with poor housing and overcrowding, and upper respiratory tract infections. In addition, the frequency of all diseases transmitted through direct person-to-person contact increases dramatically with population density; this is the case with the diseases noted above, and with measles and mumps. Weakened by malnutrition, and perhaps other diseases, children in low-income settlements often die of measles.

6. **Air.** Air pollution created by indoor fires and stoves has serious effects on the health of millions of people in the Third World. Women and children are most affected, and it is likely that high levels of air pollution in homes exacerbate respiratory illness in children. Respiratory illness, particularly among children, is one of the chief causes of mortality in the Third World.

7. **Food safety.** Apart from nutritional considerations, food can serve as a medium for the intake of toxic chemicals and microbiological agents; infections resulting from the latter are the most common type of foodborne disease. The dwellings of people in low-income groups often have few or no facilities for storing food to protect it against spoilage and contamination. Inadequate water supplies and washing facilities make the hygienic cleaning and storage of cooking utensils very difficult.

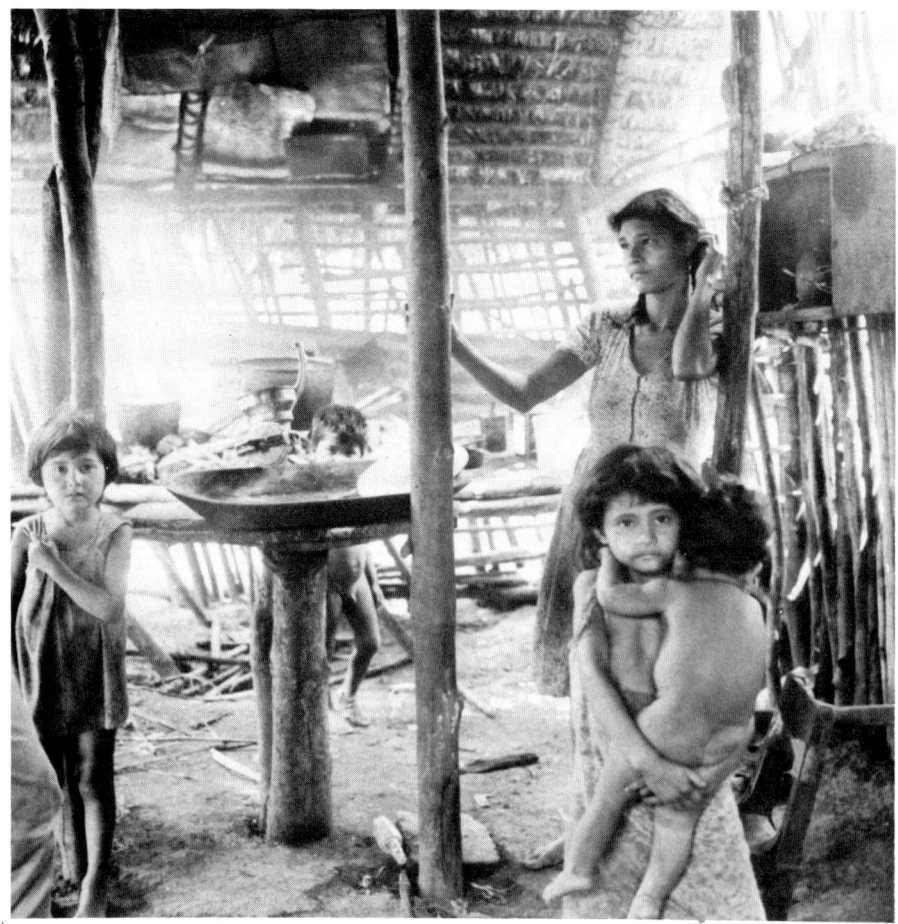

Photo WHO/P. Almasy
Poor housing conditions in parts of South America favour the spread of Chagas' disease.

8. **Vectors and hosts of disease.** Insect and animal carriers of disease present a serious problem where the climate, combined with inadequate provision for the disposal of solid wastes and wastewater, encourages the propagation of vectors. Dengue haemorrhagic fever and filariasis, spread by mosquitos, are increasing in many urban areas; onchocerciasis, schistosomiasis, and malaria, which are normally associated with rural areas, are also increasing problems in urban centres.

9. **The home as a workplace.** Using the home as a workplace can mean increased health risks from chemicals or accidents.

Without a secure home with basic services and facilities, the poor in most urban centres find their health, and indeed their survival, constantly threatened. Adults find it difficult, if not impossible, to protect their children from communicable diseases, waterborne and foodborne infections, infections spread by insanitary conditions and by intermediate animal or insect hosts, and chemical or physical hazards. The problem is all the more acute where all the adult members of a household have to work to ensure the income needed in order to survive.

Yet in the past few decades, in virtually all Third World cities, there has been a growing gap between what the poor can afford to pay for accommodation, whether bought or rented, and the cost of the cheapest accommodation that has basic services and facilities and offers its residents protection against disease or injury. On the supply side, housing prices have been pushed up by high land prices, the cost of building materials, and inappropriate building codes and land regulations. In addition, city and local governments usually lack the power and resources either to ensure a larger supply of cheap land for housing or to expand piped water, sewerage, storm drainage, and road networks to new housing developments and ensure that the inhabitants enjoy health care and emergency life-saving services. Public housing programmes have been on too small a scale to make much impact on the problem; in addition, even when subsidized, the houses that these programmes produce are too expensive for many low-income families, or ill-suited to their needs in other ways (*36, 89*). Similarly, where there are national schemes to provide health services through payments made by employers and employees, these only reach the small proportion of workers employed within formal, registered enterprises.

Only by and through government is it possible to provide facilities such as piped water, drainage and (in most instances) sanitation, garbage disposal, electricity, health care, emergency life-saving services, and education. Community or neighbourhood organizations can play a part—by, for example, helping dig drainage channels or providing volunteers to help with health education schemes—but only government can provide the city-wide framework required. Some individuals and communities are already building their own houses and planning their own settlements and, in doing so, relieving the authorities of an enormous burden.

Even a rudimentary level of environmental health cannot be achieved without public investment in the infrastructure and services desirable in all residential areas. Many low-income households cannot afford to pay the full costs of all the services and facilities required. But the real problem is rather the low priority given by the authorities to providing these services and facilities. In many instances, expenditure is concentrated on other urban investments for which there is far less social need. In addition, too little attention has been paid to collaborative schemes between government bodies and community organizations; there are a number of innovative approaches whereby government agencies can provide services and facilities in collaboration with community organizations at considerably reduced cost.[1] In the case of water supply, for example, it is often possible to install a piped system with full recovery of costs, yet charge the users less than they had previously paid to water-vendors (*14*). In addition, research encouraged by the International Drinking Water Supply and Sanitation Decade has revealed many ways in which households or communities can dispose of faecal matter at only a fraction of the cost of a sewerage system. Field studies in 39 communities in 14 countries discovered workable systems for which the annual cost per household was one-tenth to one-twentieth that of a conventional system. The cheaper systems usually needed far less water than the conventional ones, while some required no water at all. It is also possible to install one of the cheaper systems initially and then upgrade it over a period of time as the funds to do so become available (*45*).

However, city or municipal authorities tend to respond to the groups with most political and economic power and give little attention to the poor who form the majority of the urban population. In countries with large foreign debts and economies hit by the recession, problems are compounded by reductions in public expenditure. It seems likely that the next 10–20 years will bring increasing inequality to urban centres in terms of income and access to accommodation of an adequate standard with basic services and facilities.

---

[1] SHLUGER, E. *Expanding project coverage: review of urban basic services projects of Rio de Janeiro and Buenos Aires.* Paper prepared for the UNICEF Inter-regional Urban Meeting, Madras, 1987.

How the urban poor find somewhere to live

Most reports on housing problems in Third World cities state that the poor live in "slums" or "slums and shanty towns", with little indication of the various ways in which people in lower-income groups house themselves and the problems they face in doing so. The nature of these problems is often poorly understood. For instance, for the lower-income groups in any city, the location of their accommodation is often more important to their survival than its quality. A household of two adults and several children may squeeze into one room in an inner-city tenement so that the adults can be within walking distance of the main centres of employment. Better-quality accommodation may be available on the outskirts of the city, but residence there would greatly incrase the time and cost involved in getting to and from work, health care centres, and other needed services and facilities.

Above all, lower-income groups need accommodation in good locations (especially as regards access to jobs) at the lowest possible cost. Ironically, these sites are among the most expensive. Since there is often no affordable housing in a good location that meets basic needs in terms of space and services, members of lower income groups tend either to rent rooms in houses in run-down central districts, or build or rent houses or rooms in illegal housing developments on formerly unoccupied sites. Although each city will have its own unique mix of housing "submarkets" through which lower-income groups may find some form of accommodation, housing for these groups can be broken down into five broad categories; the first three are "illegal", the second two "legal".

1. Spontaneous illegal settlements: houses or shacks built by squatters on unoccupied sites, often close to the city centre, port, or business district, but also in peripheral areas.

2. Illegal settlements created by organized "invasions": houses or shacks built by squatters on land they have occupied by means of a concerted, carefully planned invasion.

3. Houses or shacks built on illegal subdivisions (i.e., subdivisions that have not had local government approval) and occupied by people who have purchased or rented them; these are usually in peripheral areas.

4. Legal rented accommodation in a central location: rented rooms in tenements, cheap boarding- or rooming-houses with high-density occupation.

5. Legal accommodation in a peripheral location: usually houses built on cheap subdivisions far enough away from centres of employment to bring down prices.

This classification is important since the means of improving environmental health will depend on the type of house, its location, and the form of tenure. Some examples of the characteristics and scale of different kinds of housing are given below; the fifth category, "Legal accommodation in a peripheral location", will not be discussed separately since the physical and environmental problems associated with this type of accommodation are usually similar to those associated with categories 1 and 3.

Spontaneous illegal settlements

Spontaneous illegal settlements can be found in most Third World cities in one form or another, wherever members of low-income groups have built houses or shacks on illegally occupied land. Once a small group of households is seen to be established on such land, others often follow. These are called by a variety of names—in Argentina, *villas miserias*; in Brazil, *favelas*; in Chile, *callampas*; in India (Delhi), *jhuggi-jhompris*; in Turkey, *gecekondus*; in Uruguay, *cantegriles*; and in Venezuela, *ranchos*.

Whatever they may be called, these settlements usually have certain physical and environmental features in common. They use illegally occupied land in a central district or on the urban periphery. Their residents are often forcefully evicted, many of them experiencing eviction from a number of different settlements in the course of their lives. Many spontaneous settlements develop on land ill-suited to housing, e.g., on hillsides prone to landslides as in Caracas, Guatemala City, La Paz, and Rio de Janeiro; on land prone to flooding or tidal inundation as in Bangkok, Bombay, Delhi, Guayaquil (Ecuador), Lagos, Monrovia, Port Moresby, and Recife (Brazil); or on sandy desert as in Khartoum and Lima. People in low-income groups choose such sites by carefully weighing up the cost, the likelihood of forceful eviction (and thus loss of the investment made in building the house), and access to employment. This accounts for the choice of dangerous or polluted sites, since these are often the cheapest and best-located sites available (*36*).

Housing and environmental conditions are usually very poor. Most settlements have little or no public provision for water supply or waste disposal. The combination of low incomes and insecure tenure often discourages investment in improvements or repairs. There is usually a high degree of overcrowding in terms of persons per room, while population density per hectare is usually high, especially in

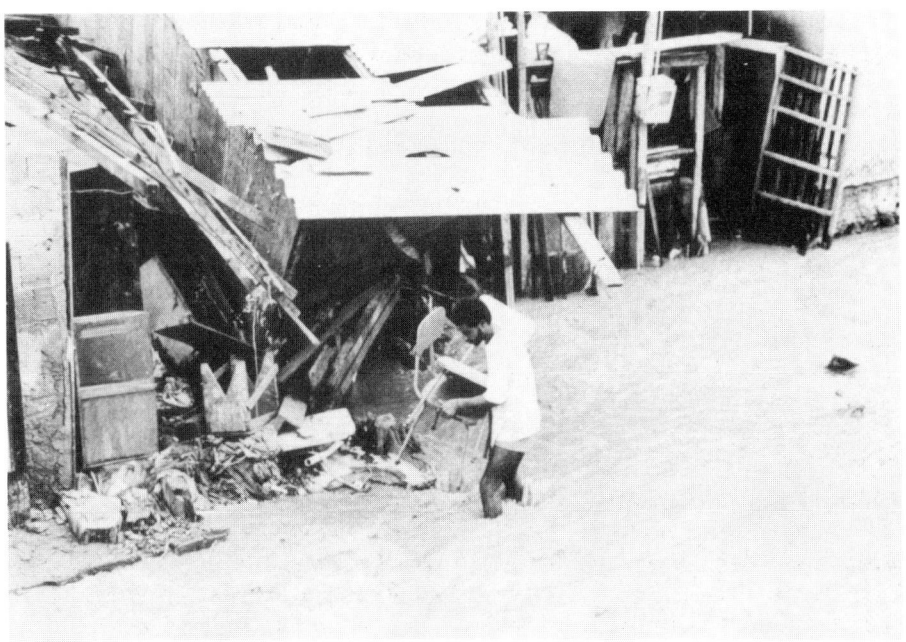

Many spontaneous settlements are built on land prone to flooding.

the older, longer established settlements. Connections to water and electricity supplies are usually illegal and precarious — or the inhabitants rely on vendors who sell water of often dubious quality at prices that can exceed by a factor of 10 or more those paid by persons in middle- or upper-income groups for piped water. Spontaneous illegal settlements have no basic plan, and thoroughfares between the houses tend to be rather small. There is little light or ventilation and often little possibility of access by vehicles in emergencies. Two-thirds of the slum population of São Paulo live in areas prone to flooding and landslides, 66% of the houses have no public lighting, 98% have no access to sewers or septic tanks, and 80% have no drinking-water (67).

Spontaneous illegal settlements often grow slowly by accretion, especially if it is seen that no steps have been taken to evict the first settlers. In the Rouse Avenue settlement next to a commercial centre in New Delhi, about 2000 people live on 1 ha of land. The first shelters were built more than 30 years ago (57). However, landowners or public authorities who have come to tolerate long-established squatters may still discourage new settlers.

Information on cities in Africa and Asia often does not distinguish between spontaneous illegal settlements, illegal subdivisions, and legal subdivisions with inadequate services and facilities. In addition, in many sub-Saharan African nations, there are settlements falling between these categories, i.e., spontaneous low-income settlements that have developed on land that is communally owned, with the approval of the person or family who traditionally had the right to allocate use of the land. Some of these settlements have been accepted by the city authorities as inevitable, so they have features of both illegal and legal subdivisions. But in virtually all instances, their inhabitants face the problems noted above, namely those arising from inadequate physical and environmental conditions and a lack of basic services and facilities.

In Bangui, Central African Republic, three-quarters of an estimated population of 340 000 (1981 figure) live in houses known as "*habitat spontané*", built by their own occupants and characterized by an absence of drinking-water supply, sanitation, and electricity. These are haphazardly distributed on land that has not been subdivided or planned, and their residents have no legal title. This situation is repeated in some of the other important cities in this country. In Nouakchott, Mauritania, an estimated 64% of the population (totalling more than 250 000 in 1982) live in largely self-built communities. More than two-thirds of the city's inhabitants have no direct access to water (*87*).

Some 38% of houses in Nairobi—estimated population in 1978, 959 000—are located in unauthorized settlements, including some on illegally invaded land, as well as irregular constructions on family plots or plots belonging to others who have allowed them to be built there. The unplanned and unauthorized settlements typically have houses built of poor-quality materials and in a poor state of repair, with little or no piped water and no sewers or drains; in addition, they lack access to roads and public lighting, and there is considerable overcrowding (*65*).

A report on Manila suggests that in 1978 there were 328 000 squatter families, totalling almost 2 million persons, living in 415 sites dotted through the urban area. This does not include the great number of people living in legal, but otherwise substandard, housing (*47*). In a report published in 1982, it was suggested that half of Delhi's population of more than 5 million were living in very poor conditions, including 700 000 people in illegal subdivisions, 600 000 or more in squatter settlements, and between 150 000 and 200 000 in what are essentially camp sites formed by squatters ejected from inner-city sites. Most of the households in each of these types of settlement have an extremely inadequate supply of water, often of poor quality, and little or no provision for sanitation, disposal of household refuse, or community services and facilities (*79a*).

These examples illustrate the common features of spontaneous illegal settlements, which stem from a total lack of the infrastructure, services, and facilities essential for health. These settlements differ considerably from one city to another in terms of security of tenure, likelihood of eviction, demographic and income structure of inhabitants, etc. But all share what has come to be termed "the environment of poverty".

Illegal settlements created by organized invasion

These have been most common in Latin America and some parts of Asia. In sharp contrast to spontaneous illegal settlements, they are highly organized, involving as they do the concerted occupation of a vacant site by large groups of households, sometimes 1000 or more. These invasions are usually carefully planned, and a site plan is worked out beforehand. They usually take place during holidays or at night and, to be able to resist eviction, as many of the invaders as possible must build temporary shelters as rapidly as they can. Some of these large-scale mobilizations of people have been accepted by governments; others have provoked a vigorous reaction from the local authorities who have tried to eject the squatters from the sites and have sometimes succeeded. Movements of this kind have been reported in Argentina, Brazil, Chile, and Peru. In all instances, the invasions were carefully organized with all the participants apparently convinced that they had a right to a piece of land on which to build, and prepared to defend this right in the courts.

Houses or shacks built on illegal subdivisions

These are often put in the same category as "spontaneous" or "squatter" settlements, although there are important differences. The most important is that the settlers have the permission of the landowner to build; the settlement is illegal not because the land is occupied illegally but because development of the site for housing has not been approved by the authorities. The inhabitants of "illegal subdivisions" are less likely to face eviction than are people living in spontaneous illegal settlements or in those formed by large organized invasions of land. But the quality of the infrastructure and services provided by the landowner or developer is usually far below the minimum standards; in many instances, no provision is made for piped water, sanitation, drainage, or paved roads. Thus, the physical and environmental problems of the inhabitants are comparable to those noted in squatter settlements.

In Calcutta, India, most of the *bustees*, in which hundreds of thousands of people live in very poor and overcrowded conditions, were originally illegal subdivisions rather than illegally occupied land. In Bogotá, a study carried out in 1973 suggested that 59% of the population were living in houses or shacks built on illegal subdivisions (so-called "pirate developments"), but that less than 1% were living in squatter settlements (*30*). In a survey of 135 "pirate" subdivisions in 1977, it was found that more than half of them lacked sewers, more than a third of them lacked water and electricity, and a fifth of them were without water, sewers, electricity, streets, or pavements (*16*).

Legal rented accommodation with a central location

This type of accommodation is common throughout the Third World and in many parts of developed countries. It usually consists of individual rooms let out to households or groups of individuals with bathroom, laundry, and kitchen facilities shared between 30 or more people. It includes tenements and cheap boarding- and rooming-houses. In most instances, the buildings were subdivided when the middle- or upper-income groups for whom they were originally intended moved out to the suburbs. Thus, they were never meant to house the number of people who live in them now; ten or more families may be living in quarters originally designed for one or two. Tenements are usually neglected and in a poor state of repair.

In Latin America, tenements developed as a major urban feature during periods of heavy international migration, mainly at the end of the nineteenth century. In many countries, tenements are chosen by individuals or households in the lower-income groups because they are well located in relation to the city centre, access to work, and public service facilities such as schools and hospitals. For the owners of these buildings, the high rents (relative to the services provided) make them equally attractive, even though this has done nothing to encourage building maintenance or improvements in services (*75*). It is estimated that, in the metropolitan area of Guatemala, 60% of the total housing available consists of tenements. In Delhi, almost 1.3 million people live in tenements (*57*), and in Guayaquil, Ecuador, 250 000 people were estimated to be living in them in 1980 (*77*). However, their inner city location often makes tenement buildings attractive to property developers for redevelopment, either as offices or business premises or as flats for people in the middle- or upper-income groups. In many places, the availability of cheap accommodation for rent in central districts is declining as a result, although new rental markets are growing rapidly in many of the better located squatter settlements and illegal subdivisions, and in areas where tenements have not traditionally been concentrated. It should be noted that the demographic structure of tenement districts may differ considerably from the city norm in ways that have important implications for health; surveys in the central areas of certain Latin American cities recorded a substantially higher-than-average number of people over 60 years of age. Many older people living in city centres are trapped in tenements because of inadequate pensions or inability to find employment providing a reasonable income (*34, 35*).

3
Neighbourhood organizations and health

How and why neighbourhood organizations are formed

The concentration of people in urban centres where there is little or no provision for piped water, sanitation, and other essential services and facilities has given rise to community- or neighbourhood-based organizations or associations of residents, whose aim is to try to improve living conditions.

The diversity of cities in terms of scale and structure, as noted in the Introduction, is reflected in the many forms taken by the organizations set up by the residents. The form they take, the issues around which they are organized, and the way in which they are organized differ greatly from place to place. However, experience in Latin America suggests that in all types of low-income settlement, from spontaneous squatter settlements to organized invasions and illegal subdivisions, neighbourhood organizations of some kind usually develop. These include neighbourhood committees or councils, promotion societies, mothers' unions, and teenage associations. In neighbourhoods with a high proportion of rented accommodation, tenants' associations may be set up. In some cities, neighbourhood committees or councils join with similar organizations to form federations.

Despite the different forms taken by these organizations and the different names they adopt, most of them are created to provide a concrete collective response to a problem facing or affecting a substantial number of the people in a neighbourhood. In virtually every instance, these problems are related either to environmental health or to security of tenure. In respect of environmental health, neighbourhood organizations are often set up in response to the inadequate provision of such amenities as water supply, all-weather access roads and paths, rain- and stormwater drainage, hygienic removal of household and human wastes, and electricity, or to some special health threat to the settlement (e.g., from flooding, landslides, or high levels of air or water pollution). In respect of security of tenure, they may be organized either to help members acquire land on which to build, or to help protect members from eviction. If members' houses are built on illegally occupied land, neighbourhood associations may organize to fight eviction or to negotiate with the public authorities and landowners to acquire secure tenure. If members are tenants, their interests are likely to be centred on tenants' rights.

Perhaps the most common kind of neighbourhood organization is one set up to tackle a specific problem; for instance, in squatter settlements in Greater Buenos Aires, work groups are formed to dig and maintain drainage ditches to prevent flooding and help dispose of wastewater (*32*). Also common is the setting up of some service — for instance, communal nurseries or day-care programmes organized by women to allow them to undertake full-time or part-time work. Sports clubs and teenage associations are also common in low-income settlements (*98*). These organizations may grow out of smaller, more informal arrangements through which neighbours help one another: as Guber (*32*) noted in Buenos Aires, people in squatter settlements may allow neighbours to use a private water-tap or bathroom; similarly, they may keep an eye on neighbours' houses when they are out, take care of each other's children, or exchange essential items such as matches, fat for cooking, flour, needles, or yarn.

Sometimes the main role of a neighbourhood organization is to petition the city or municipal authority to provide some service — for instance, piped water or a school. This type of organization is often relatively complex, with leaders acknowledged as having the contacts or organizational skills required to negotiate with public agencies. There are also examples of neighbourhood organizations formed by squatters who have successfully negotiated with landowners and public authorities to acquire legal ownership of the sites on which their houses or shacks are built; in the city of Bangkok, "land-sharing" agreements have been reached between landowners and community organizations whereby landowners receive part of the site in return for the granting of legal tenure to all those living on the other part (S. Angel & S. Boonyabancha, unpublished information, 1985).

Some studies suggest that neighbourhood organizations originally set up to initiate or manage communal work, or provide a service, often develop into pressure groups that lobby city or municipal governments to provide basic services (*81*). Neighbourhood-based organizations have often joined forces, since this can make them more effective in negotiations with public agencies. Some may acquire legal status with defined objectives, rules, and internal structures; these are usually found where the inhabitants have acquired legal tenure of their houses.

In Latin America, it is common for women to play the major role in neighbourhood organizations, even if men figure as the leaders or spokesmen. This was the situation observed by Moser (*61*) in Guayaquil, Ecuador's largest city, where more than half the population live in squatter settlements built on stilts over a tidal swamp, with most houses reached by narrow catwalks: "Women living in the same street are constantly thrown together; when the water tanker fails to arrive, they stand in groups discussing how to share what they have; when a child is killed falling off the catwalks, women gather to console a grieving neighbour . . . through interaction of this kind they become aware that the problem is not simply an individual one but common to all women." Usually, it is women who take the primary responsibility for nursing babies and looking after children, in addition to domestic chores (including fetching water)—not to mention nursing sick members of the family, even though they themselves may also be in paid employment. It is they who are most affected by their families' needs and deprivations.

The form that a neighbourhood organization takes will naturally be greatly influenced by the neighbourhood in which it develops. Many neighbourhood organizations develop when the population is already settled; for instance, a settlement that takes shape slowly on illegal subdivisions is unlikely at first to have such well organized neighbourhood associations as one based on a large-scale land invasion. In most such invasions, the level of organization was generally already high before the invasion took place. Indeed this is what ensured the successful large-scale settlement of the areas invaded. But whatever form they take, neighbourhood organizations and the wider "popular movements" fostered by the representatives of such organizations have become highly influential in some cities and are likely to become increasingly important in many others. This is especially so in cities where the incomes of an increasing proportion of the population are not enough to meet the cost of basic items such as food, clothing, transport, water, and health care.

Three case studies from Latin America

In São Paulo, Brazil, Latin America's second largest city (with a population of some 12.6 million in the metropolitan area in 1980), numerous neighbourhood movements have developed since the early 1970s to tackle problems of environmental health and press for better health care services. For example, in 1979, in Jardin Nordeste, a health council representing more than 8000 residents was elected. A commission of 12 women was elected with the initial task of supervising the functioning of the health centre. They held street meetings at which complaints were collected to be passed on to the Secretariat for Health. Here, the impetus for neighbourhood organization was provided by the inadequacy of the health services. As Jacobi noted in 1983 (*44*):

> In the health centres of São Paulo there is a lack of physicians, officials, powdered milk and even hygiene . . . Problems start in the early morning hours with long lines in the middle of the street and fights for consultation tags. Consultations are due to start at 7 a.m. but do not start until 8 . . . the physician receives 15 patients per day between former and new patients, as well as emergencies, and then leaves. The people know it is not his fault. A doctor who works there has to be some sort of hero because if he is a sensitive person he will suffer more than the patient. Doctors in these dispensaries spend practically all their wages on transportation because in general they live far away. Furthermore, they need a second job which makes their work even more difficult.

Among the catalysts of this neighbourhood action were outbreaks of measles and other diseases which resulted in the death of several children for want of adequate medical help. These led to the development of the health commission consisting of people from the neighbourhood who, after one year of lobbying, had a health centre installed on rented premises. Later, they succeeded in electing a new council. All this encouraged the people living in the neighbourhood to attend, and make use of, the health centre.

The organization then widened its objectives to tackle the health problems evident in the living environment:

> In time, the health council achieved certain success and the people became aware of other problems in the neighbourhood (and there were many) and decided that maybe these could be solved in the same way. So other commissions were created for transportation, nurseries, pavements, culture, subdivisions, until finally the 'Movement for better living standards in Jardin Nordeste' was formed. This movement has no relationship — as their members point out — with any other agency, nor with the Church, the Societies of Friends of the Neighbourhood, or political parties, even if they all coexist peacefully together.

In Santiago, the capital of Chile, it was again the need for health services that prompted neighbourhood action; this, too, widened to encompass environmental improvements. In the Raul Silva Henriquez and Juan Francisco Frenso *campamentos*, organizations formed by the squatter inhabitants approached various groups to get help in improving conditions. In the area of health, help was provided by the Church, the medical school, the Association of Young Physicians, and medical students. But one of the key factors in what proved to be successful action for better health was the inhabitants' own organization. The settlement was divided into sections, and a health delegate was chosen from each section to represent it in the Health Brigade. A Health Manager was appointed to coordinate activities. This set-up permitted the monitoring and control of health risks (for instance, outbreaks of disease) and the organization of training seminars and courses on first aid, disease prevention, and the control of infectious and parasitic diseases. A health workshop monitored work already completed and proposed new lines of action (*40*).

> The three main [health] problems which needed the attention of social workers (monitors) for all age groups were respiratory diseases, diarrhoea and wounds. The former two have consistently decreased from January to October, a fact perhaps due to better climatic conditions and some improvement in the dwellings. The trend towards a noticeable decrease in diarrhoea could be ascribed to the installation of running water in the month of December. In both cases, as well as for wounds, training and sanitary education may have been instrumental.

Action was also taken to tackle other environmental problems: refuse disposal, care of domestic animals, and food preparation. Urgent housing problems were also tackled through a team of architects and squatters, whose activities included site planning and the construction of communal showers and sinks. In addition, legal action was taken to establish the inhabitants' right to have medical centres provided for them by the Government, and, after substantial lobbying, this too proved successful.

In Buenos Aires, the San Martin *barrio* in the municipality of Quilmes was formed by means of a large-scale invasion of vacant land in 1981. The site had no water supply, sewers, or storm-/rainwater drainage. Despite the fact that the occupation of the land was illegal — and initially strongly resisted by the (then) military government — the inhabitants planned the layout of the site in such a way as to leave enough space for access roads and community facilities. While, at that time, the public authorities ignored the inhabitants' request for water, electricity, and health care, the government elected in 1983 has proved more sympathetic to squatters' needs, both at national and at local (municipal) level.

Initially, the inhabitants' three most pressing needs were electricity, water, and health care. Illegal connections to existing electricity and water systems met the first two needs — though inadequately. In 1983, as political parties became more active in the run-up to the elections, a neighbourhood coordinating committee began negotiations with each party to try to ensure that basic services would be provided and their tenure of the land legalized. These negotiations met with little success initially. So, supported by the local priest and sympathetic professional health workers, the community organized a very basic system of health care and health information for themselves. The outbreaks of diarrhoea each summer did much to stimulate these initiatives. Although neighbourhood action for health varied in strength and effectiveness, it did finally result in the construction of a health care centre. In mid-1983, the neighbourhood committee offered what was in effect a symbolic wage to a doctor who had volunteered to help. Fees were collected from the inhabitants, and the centre was constructed. In the organizational tasks, including running the dispensary, women have usually played the major role (*24*).

4
The role of local government

Local government and health

Although the form taken by local government differs widely from one country to another — as does its relationship with higher levels of government and specialized agencies, and the division of resources and responsibilities among them — it remains the level of government from which the cheapest, most effective public initiatives to tackle problems of child health can be launched. This is the case whether its jurisdiction is city-wide or, as is the case in many larger cities or metropolitan areas, covers only one part of the city.

City or municipal authorities have most of the legal and institutional responsibility for the planning and maintenance of the urban area under their jurisdiction and for ensuring that those living there are provided with services and facilities: water, sanitation, disposal of solid wastes, electricity, drainage, paved roads and pathways, etc. They are usually responsible for providing schools, hospitals and health care centres, and emergency life-saving services. They are usually entrusted with the control of new residential developments, ensuring, for instance, that the services and facilities provided are of an adequate standard and that the buildings meet health and safety standards.

Local government is also the level of government best equipped to assess and understand local needs and mobilize local resources to deal with such needs. As Julius Nyerere, the then President of the United Republic of Tanzania, commented in 1972:

> Our nation is too large for the people at the centre in Dar es Salaam always to understand local problems or sense their urgency. When all the power remains at the centre, therefore, local problems can remain and fester, while local people who are aware of them are prevented from using their initiative in finding solutions . . . at present (local) officials have, in reality, very little local power. They have to consult the Ministries in Dar es Salaam for almost everything they wish to do and certainly about every cent they wish to spend.

Nevertheless it is with government at the city or municipal level that the urban dweller must deal. While national ministries or agencies can play very important supporting and advisory roles, action at neighbourhood level to tackle problems of health, including child health, must be locally formulated and implemented, otherwise it will not respond to local needs and build on local resources and capabilities.

It is thus particularly important to strengthen the capacity of local government, which, in most developing countries, lacks the power, resources, and trained personnel to meet the responsibilities outlined above. As a report by the World Bank recently noted, many local authorities are "fragmented, confused about their functions and all too often either invisible or largely ceremonial" (23). Local government is the only institution that can provide the planning, coordination, and institutional structure required to implement the two most important policy initiatives recommended in the World Bank report: a large increase in official recognition of, and support for, the role of neighbourhood associations in tackling health problems, and a higher priority, at the national government level, to the allocation of resources to agencies or ministries concerned with public works that promote environmental health, such as water supply, sanitation, and drainage schemes, or concerned with preventive health or health care.

At present, most city and municipal governments lack either the funding or the revenue-raising power to permit investment in improving or even maintaining environmental health. Even in urban centres with rapidly growing populations, and thus with rapidly growing needs for piped water, sanitation, drainage, etc., local government usually has little or no investment capacity. Typically, in the countries concerned, the national governments receive much higher proportions of taxes and other revenues than is usual in "western" nations, and the ratio of government employees in agencies or ministries at the national level to those in local government is much higher. Argentina provides a good example. In 1975, the central government received an income equivalent to 7.7% of the gross national product (GNP), while, in the same year, all the local authorities in the country only received 0.7%. In 1980, the central government received 11.3% of the GNP, and the local authorities 0.9%. Finally, in 1985, the central government received 13.8% of the GNP, and the local authorities 1.1% (17). Comparable statistics could be quoted for many other countries.

City, municipal, and departmental authorities are not only without resources of their own, but have lost the capacity to raise the funds they need by means of loans or credits, which are concentrated at national level. For instance, in Colombia in 1981, total internal and external credits were distributed in the following way: the national government received 79.4%, the departments 7.3%, and the municipalities 13.3%. The last mentioned allocation went mostly to the provincial capitals. In addition, the central government received almost 85% of all income from taxes (*79*).

Thus, a lack of resources is forcing local authorities either to cut down on the provision (or maintenance) of services or to hand over the responsibility to provincial, regional, or national organizations. Above all, the key to dealing with child health problems in urban areas is a local authority that understands the needs of the local population and has the resources to meet them. This suggests new roles and directions for international aid. Official multilateral and bilateral aid is channelled through central governments; where this aid is provided in the form of a loan (whether on commercial or concessional terms), it is central government that has to guarantee repayment. "Moreover, until recently, aid agencies did not often concern themselves with the problems of municipal administration: such problems are still given low priority. Significantly, three recent World Bank publications make no mention of local government or administration and its role in implementing urbanisation policies" (*57*). However, the increasing emphasis placed by the World Bank and certain other aid agencies on building the institutional capacity of city and municipal governments and increasing their revenue base is a recognition that improvements in the health and housing of urban populations depend to a large extent on more effective action at the local government level.

Financial weakness is also responsible for the low technical level of local administrations, from both a qualitative and a quantitative standpoint. In general, there has been a weakening of local government in almost all Third World Countries, as a result of the increased centralization of decisions and powers by most of the national governments.

Local government and neighbourhood associations

Given the limited amount of funds available to local (and often national) authorities, and the time needed to strengthen the powers of local government, the most promising and cost-effective approach for government action is an alliance between local government and neighbourhood organizations. The three case studies outlined in Chapter 3 (page 46) give some idea of the potential for action offered by neighbourhood organizations, given appropriate public support.

There are also some precedents on which to build. One of the best known is furnished by the city of Hyderabad, India, where the municipal corporation set up an Urban Community Development Department to work in direct liaison with community groups and nongovernmental organizations operating in low-income neighbourhoods. This agency responds to the needs expressed by local residents, rather than offering some predetermined package of public investments and interventions.[1] In addition, most of the squatter settlements that have developed on government land have been "regularized", i.e., their inhabitants granted legal tenure. Another example comes from Mexico, where in 1981 the Federal Government set up a National Fund for Popular Housing which provides credits to cooperatives and other legally constituted groups organized by the inhabitants of low-income settlements, and to local authorities.

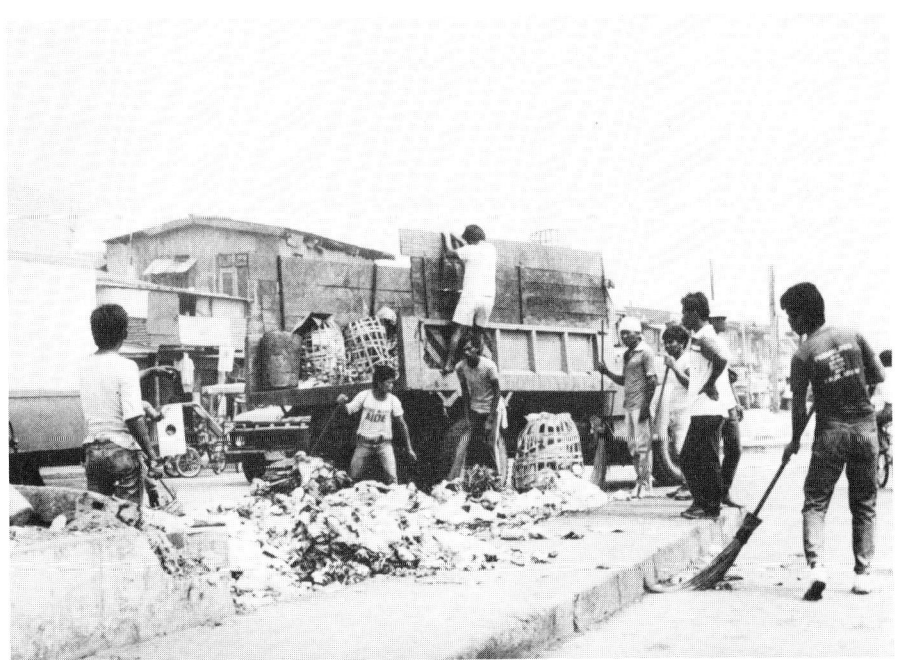

Photo WHO/E. Ouano

Local residents help an undermanned garbage collection unit to clean up the area.

---

[1] UNITED NATIONS CENTRE FOR HUMAN SETTLEMENTS (HABITAT). *Hyderabad squatter settlement upgrading project, India*. Nairobi, 1986 (Project monograph produced for the International Year of Shelter for the Homeless).

The Hyderabad example also provides insights into the initiation of the type of action required. For example, low-income groups and their organizations knew what they needed but were less clear on how to achieve their objectives:

> They did not know how to draw up petitions about local needs or improvements and submit them to the relevant departments. Within a short time, rubbish was cleared and dustbins that had been badly located were shifted to better places upon the recommendations of local residents ... and one slum community which had received no piped water was provided with a connection from a nearly housing colony where all the houses had individual water taps.[1]

The example also shows that members of the community are the best people to identify the means by which objectives can most appropriately be attained.

Another good example of a dialogue between a community and the local authority is the upgrading programme in the Rocinha district of Rio de Janeiro, Brazil, on which a city-wide programme was subsequently based. Rocinha, one of Rio's largest and longest established *favelas*, has 80 000 inhabitants, over half of them under 14 years of age. During the rainy season, accumulations of raw sewage and garbage from every part of the settlement used to be washed down, along with domestic wastewater, in open drains. These drains often flooded the lowest-lying areas — which were also the poorest.

There is a long history of community activity within Rocinha. For example, a *mutirao* (mutual aid group) was set up by residents in 1970 to clean public areas and clear ditches on Sundays and holidays, the basic tools for these tasks being supplied by the local authorities. With time, services in the settlement have improved; there are now 3 day-care centres, 3 health posts, and 2 community schools run and supported by the residents. The inhabitants have formed health and sanitation groups and cooperated with the municipal authorities in a scheme to improve the main sewage ditch. When a lack of external funds threatened the continuity of the programme, the mutual aid group merged with the sanitation group to strengthen their bargaining power with the public authorities and to increase their capacity to implement action for development.

In 1979, these groups, together with a new Municipal Secretariat for Social Development and local UNICEF staff, started a project to

---

[1] RAO, R. *Urban community development project—Hyderabad.* Paper presented at workshop organized by OXFAM, UNICEF, and the London School of Hygiene and Tropical Medicine, 7–12 July 1985.

upgrade the *favela*. They began with a survey to provide the information on which to base their programme, which sought at the outset to promote water supply, sanitation, informal education, and health services. In 1982, a demonstration project was started in Rocinha, which was selected because of the high level of organization prevailing there. It received the support of local leaders and members of the residents' sanitation group. Other residents were paid to work part-time to ensure liaison between residents and engineers and to help mobilize residents for construction work. The project concentrated on completing work on the sewerage system and on measures such as drainage, paving the area around the water-tap, and constructing a collection-point for garbage cans. A seminar was held beforehand to allow staff from government agencies to discuss aspects of public policy for the *favela* areas with members of the community.

When, in 1982, the municipal authorities announced their plans to extend the programme to other *favelas*, 60 *favelas* asked to be included. However, because of technical and financial constraints, only 9 of them could be selected for "Project Mutirao" which nevertheless resulted in construction work benefiting some 18 000 people and costing less than half of what it would have cost if entrusted to an ordinary contractor. It is estimated that the residents absorbed around 25% of the cost of purchasing the materials used. Early in 1986, there were plans to extend the project to 96 *favelas* (*13, 19*).[1]

The task facing both national and urban governments is to make initiatives of this kind the norm rather than the exception. This means that city and municipal governments will have to recognize the health needs of all those within their jurisdiction. In the past, they have often proved reluctant to do so, especially in the case of people living in illegal settlements, even where these represent half or more of the population of their jurisdiction and include a large part of the labour force and the businesses that make up the local cconomy. It is still common for squatters not to figure in population statistics, since they are not regarded as official city residents by the authorities (*9*).

The illegal status of many low-income settlements makes local governments reluctant to work with their neighbourhood associations, since that would implicitly acknowledge their right to

---

[1] SHLUGER, E. *Expanding project coverage: review of urban basic services projects of Rio de Janeiro and Buenos Aires.* Paper prepared for the UNICEF Inter-regional Urban Meeting, Madras, 1987.

municipal services. As a result, the authorities are largely unfamiliar with the problems of those living in the settlements. If people feel that there is little possibility of receiving some publicly funded services, this in turn inhibits the formation and development of strong neighbourhood-based organizations. The strength and potential impact of such bodies is very much linked to the inhabitants' perceptions of what can be achieved by working together.

One result of the lack of knowledge, on the part of local government, about conditions in low-income settlements is almost certainly that the scale of their health problems is considerably underestimated. It is common to find broad comparisons made between mortality indicators for "urban" and "rural" areas which show that the urban areas generally have lower infant and child mortality rates. Such comparisons may be very misleading. Firstly, averages "for all urban areas", or for one city in particular, appear low because a high proportion of middle- and upper-income groups live in cities — and are provided with piped water, sewers, drains, and emergency life-saving services, as well as having access to health care. Case studies already cited suggest that infant and child mortality rates (and other indicators of health status) may be worse in squatter communities or inner-city tenements than in "rural areas". Indeed, another reason why official health surveys may seem to suggest that urban dwellers have better health could be that people living in squatter settlements are not covered by them. As Rossi-Espagnet has pointed out, "a systematic study of intra-urban differentials in health and health-related conditions has not been carried out anywhere in the developing world".[1] Indeed, to work out whether infant and child health problems are concentrated in "urban" or in "rural" areas may be a useless exercise. The important thing is to identify the groups with the most serious health problems and those that are most vulnerable; these are likely to be more closely correlated with levels of income, gender, age, and occupation than with whether the groups are "rural" or "urban". What is likely to emerge is that too little attention has been paid to the environmental health problems of low-income groups in urban centres.

Confronting the problem as a whole

It is now well accepted that "health is the responsibility of the individual, the community and the government as a whole" and "is therefore ultimately a political question. . . . In certain countries significant changes in health will be possible only through funda-

---

[1] ROSSI-ESPAGNET, A. *Primary health care in urban areas: reaching the urban poor in developing countries. A state-of-the-art report.* Unpublished UNICEF/WHO document, SHS 84.4.

mental social and economic change" (5). The very poor quality of life shared by most of the urban poor in Third World countries — with their high levels of infant and child mortality and morbidity — is likewise a product of their social and economic status.

If the level of their health is to be raised, political decisions will be needed about priorities in the allocation of resources for the improvement of housing and the residential environment (covering such aspects as water and sanitation, drainage, safe, secure and affordable land sites for new housing, and garbage disposal), together with efficient preventive services (covering vaccination and immunization, maternity and child welfare, and health education) and health care services. There is little point in improving the quality of care for cases of infant and child diarrhoea, or running a programme to teach primary school children personal hygiene, if the contaminated drinking-water or living environment that makes reinfection virtually certain is not dealt with. Indeed, medical care services would be overloaded if their improvement did not go hand-in-hand with improvements in preventive health measures and the physical environment.

To ensure improvements in housing and the residential environment, including the provision of basic services, national governments will have to build up the capacity and competence of local authorities. As noted earlier, only governments at city, municipal, or district level are in a position to install, extend, and maintain the requisite services and facilities, and to forge successful relationships with neighbourhood associations, as described in the previous chapter. In the light of severe shortages of public funds, the second consideration is as important as the first, since the cooperation envisaged permits limited resources to be used to maximum effect.

In many cities, nongovernmental organizations are already deeply involved in tackling the environmental health problems of lower income groups. Such organizations were responsible for many of the studies — noted earlier — showing the magnitude of the health problems confronting the groups in question and the extent to which they were linked to poor housing and lack of basic services and facilities. Building up a stable and effective long-term relationship between local government and community and neighbourhood associations in order to tackle housing and environmental health problems takes time. Nongovernmental organizations can often form an important link between them, helping local authorities with needed research and giving them appropriate technical advice. This is particularly the case when they already have experience both in research (through working with lower-income groups in identifying major health problems and their causes) and in action (through providing community groups with technical and legal advice and developing infrastructure).

A comprehensive health policy, as proposed in the Alma-Ata Declaration (71), implies that local authorities should have a good knowledge of health problems and how they change over time. At present, very few of them do. This knowledge must be built up, along with the necessary institutional structure, so that their measures to improve the health of lower income groups may be taken in full awareness of the problems and priorities of these groups. Indeed, the fewer resources available, the more important the need for accurate knowledge about the principal health problems and their causes so that these resources may be used to maximum effect.

Improvements in knowledge and the establishment of relationships with community associations will call the traditional patterns of expenditure on health and health care into question, especially the priority given to conventional hospital-based, curative health care systems (22). Investment in piped water, rain- and stormwater drainage, and systems for the hygienic disposal of household and human wastes in urban areas is likely to prove far more effective in improving the health of the inhabitants than investment in new hospitals. Research undertaken in Argentina in the early 1970s confirmed that improved housing conditions and the provision of basic services led to more dramatic improvements in the health status of lower-income urban groups than investments in traditional hospital-based medical care (8).

The need for an approach to health care that stresses improvements in housing and the residential environment, and preventive measures as well as medical facilities, has become widely accepted since it was spelt out at the Alma-Ata Conference in 1978 (71). However, governments and the relevant institutions have been slow to make the necessary changes. An additional problem is that professional health workers are largely geared to curative medicine rather than preventive measures or the promotion of health-enhancing behaviour; in addition, their education has not equipped them with the knowledge and skills required in order to work with the people who have the most serious health problems and are in most need of professional advice, care, and support (43).

Official figures on the distribution of professional health workers can be very misleading. Judgements about the extent to which a population is served are often made on the basis of statistics aggregated in such a way as to hide the real situation. To take but one example, the city of Buenos Aires appears to be well served with physicians, since there is one for every 200 inhabitants. In the

Province of Buenos Aires, however, which includes a very substantial proportion of the population of Metropolitan Buenos Aires, there are 1.7 physicians per 1000 inhabitants and, at the periphery of the city, where the most economically disadvantaged groups live, there is an acute shortage of physicians.[1]

Official statistics concerning the location and utilization of facilities may also obscure, rather than clarify, health problems. There may, for example, appear to be enough dispensaries, health care centres, or hospitals at the city or municipal level, if one ignores the fact that large sections of the population live in areas from which it is difficult, expensive, and time-consuming to reach them. Or perhaps the opening hours of these facilities are inconvenient for many low-income households. The fact that all the adult members of many of these households work full-time means that it is difficult for them to visit these facilities on their own account, or bring their children to them, unless they are open outside normal working hours, which is rarely the case. Special problems of access to health care arise in the case of households headed by women, where the head of the household has to fulfil the triple role of main income-earner, child-rearer, and housekeeper.

Even when the facilities are close at hand, people in low-income groups may still receive very inadequate health care. For instance, the inhabitants of Chheetpur in Allahabad, India, whose health problems have already been described, have a hospital that provides free health care within a kilometre of their homes. But they complain that they have to queue for hours before receiving treatment and then they are often told that, for proper treatment, they would have to come to the doctor's own private clinic, where, of course, they would have to pay (59). In other surveys of health service utilization, it has been shown that understaffing, inadequate supplies of medicines and of other necessary goods or equipment, and long queues present problems for people in lower-income groups. Another problem, highlighted by Lapaco (personal communication) is the lack of continuity created by changes in government commitments as a result of which health care services in a low-income community or area may be suddenly discontinued; people's faith in such services quickly vanishes if they are not seen to answer their needs.

There is also the difficulty of matching the sheer complexity of the factors impinging on the health status of infants, children, and

---

[1] BIANCO, M. *Health and its care in greater Buenos Aires.* Paper presented at the Joint UNICEF/WHO Meeting on Primary Health Care in Urban Areas, Geneva, July 1983.

adults with the sectoral and often simplistic programmes or projects that are meant to improve health. According to unpublished information from Raczynski on the effects of the recent economic recession on infant health in Chile, malnutrition has been increasing among children as a result of need at home and inadequate nutrition programmes at school. Although the information the author furnishes is incomplete, it is nevertheless consistent. A survey carried out in poor areas of the *comuna* of San Miguel, within the metropolitan area of Santiago, Chile, showed an increase in malnutrition among schoolchildren between 1980 and 1983. The proportion of schoolchildren suffering from malnutrition, calculated on the basis of the FAO/WHO criteria using weight-to-height ratios, increased from 4.6% to 15.8%. One of the problems that can be inferred from programmes of the type described is that it is unclear whether school meals represented the children's only energy intake or whether they were complemented by other meals or snacks. The sole criterion available for assessing the distribution of family meals (said to cover only 33% of the daily energy requirements established by FAO and WHO) seems to have been the personal evaluation of the schoolteacher.

In such circumstances, the possibility of using the administrative structure responsible for the programme to generate precise information vanishes. With appropriate short training courses, backed up by manuals, schoolteachers could become a most important source of information (and act as monitors) of children's health and nutritional status, quite apart from the important part they can play in health education. Similarly, other professional people whose work brings them into direct contact with the inhabitants of low-income settlements — especially people who make house calls, such as midwives and nurses — could also help provide the type of information needed to bring about a better understanding by the authorities of the health problems of the urban poor.

It is essential to realize that, in the precarious settlements concerned, one sectoral action or programme dealing with health or housing cannot by itself have more than a limited impact on infant and child health. This is a point that has been well established by studies, including many of those already mentioned. For water and sanitation, as Elmendorf & Isely (*29*) point out, the experiences in recent projects point to the need for careful consideration of local conditions, practices, preferences and beliefs. This implies the need to involve fully the people for whom the improvements are intended in planning, implementation and evaluation. Since women are major users of water, as well as educators of children about hygiene and use of toilets, their participation is particularly critical. It is all the more so where, as is commonly the case, they also have responsibilities for managing and maintaining facilities. Ignoring such issues when installing new water or sanitation systems has often led to breakdown of the systems with no one having the knowledge or motivation to repair them. "It has been found that 35–50% of systems in many developing countries become inoperable after five years" (*29*).

One final point concerns "street children". A considerable proportion of children in the towns and cities of developing countries spend much of their lives on the streets, trying to earn some money. During the current recession and the debt crisis prevailing in most of these countries, the number of street children has increased very considerably. Most of them have homes to return to at the end of the day and the pressures pushing them on to the street are created simply by the inability of their families to earn enough through the efforts of their adult members alone.

The need to contribute to the family income often means that children's schooling is curtailed so that they can work. To give just two examples of the scale of child labour: in Ecuador over 30% of children are engaged in some form of work (*86*) while in Bogotá, the capital of Colombia, 87% of the primary schoolchildren from the lowest-income groups regularly work in family or other businesses or do housework (*10*). Most earning opportunities for children are to be found on the street, although they may also be employed in factories, workshops, and shops at very low wages. The root cause of their presence on the street is the same as the root cause of poor housing and undernutrition, i.e., inadequate earning opportunities. Little more than a century ago, the phenomenon of "street children" and the widespread exploitation of child labour were major problems throughout the rapidly urbanizing "western" world. They are unlikely to decline much in the Third World, unless — as in the West — poverty itself declines.

In many cities, some street children have only tenuous ties with their family or no ties with them at all. While these seem to constitute only a small proportion of all street children, their numbers can nevertheless run into thousands and perhaps even tens of thousands in some of the larger metropolitan areas. Again, poverty is the root cause. Abandoned or street children are especially vulnerable to abuse and exploitation. Lacking education and competing with adults for very limited earning opportunities, their strategies for survival often involve illegal acts. Urgent action is needed to provide children who have no family home with a stable, safe place to live in, and with education and training. Urgent action is also needed to help children from low-income households, since it is these children who are most likely to leave home permanently.

Here, as in most areas requiring urgent action, it is difficult to be specific, since the scale and nature of the problem vary so much from city to city. What is needed is the strengthening of the capacity of local government to assess the scale and nature of the problem and to take appropriate action, making the best possible use of local resources.

5
Summary, conclusions, and recommendations

Earlier chapters have indicated the vast scale on which ill health and premature deaths occur among lower-income groups in the urban centres of the Third World. They have shown how most of the areas where they live have little or no provision for piped water, sanitation, the removal of household wastes, storm- and surface-water drainage, paved roads, or an electricity supply. Most cities in developing countries have no sewerage system at all, or, if they do, it serves only a small part of the city. Their water supply systems reach only a small proportion of the population and lack the capacity to meet even minimum water requirements for most of their inhabitants. Virtually all local government authorities in urban areas lack the investment capacity to extend piped water, sewers, paved roads, and drainage systems to all residential areas. When this situation is combined with overcrowding and often with insecure tenure, it contributes greatly to ill health and premature death.

As a rule, infants and children are those most affected, since they spend most time in and near the home and are particularly vulnerable to the health hazards found there: communicable diseases, water- and foodborne infections, diseases spread by poor sanitary conditions and intermediate insect or animal hosts, chemical hazards from air, water, and soil pollution, and physical hazards from floods, fires, and traffic. The environment within which hundreds of millions of children grow and develop is not conducive to either their physical or their mental development.

In "western" nations, most of the environmental health hazards associated with urban living have been greatly reduced by means of better-quality housing with adequate services and facilities. This is a result both of much higher purchasing power on the part of the population (so that better-quality housing could be paid for) and of a government structure able to raise revenue and invest in the requisite services and facilities in each urban centre. Higher incomes have also improved people's diets so that the problem of children's defences against infection being weakened by malnutrition has been much reduced. Although housing problems still exist in many countries in the northern hemisphere and affect the health of people in lower-income groups, their scale and the proportion of people they affect are of a different order of magnitude from those obtaining in virtually all Third World countries. The basic investment in water systems, sewers, drains, roads, health care, and preventive services and facilities has been made, even if funds are now needed to improve or maintain them. In addition, the structures of city and municipal government and the public recognition of the role and responsibilities of government in protecting citizens from the health hazards inherent in poor housing and living environments have been realities for decades.

The task facing governments of developing countries is threefold: as a matter of high priority, to tackle the very serious health problems confronting many of their population through multisectoral action to improve housing and the residential environment, provide basic amenities, improve the nutritional level of the population, and organize basic preventive health, health care, and emergency life-saving services; to build up the administrative structures required for these purposes at city and district level; and to obtain the capital to pay for the necessary basic urban infrastructure.

Urgent action is needed now. In many Third World countries, a child born today is 15–20 times more likely to die before the age of 5 than a child born in a prosperous "western" nation. In many squatter settlements where there is no public provision for water supply, sanitation, household waste collection or health care, a child born today is 40–50 times more likely to die before the age of 5 than a child born in a prosperous nation. In virtually all developing countries, the majority of infant and child deaths are preventable at relatively low cost. So too are most of the diseases and accidents that continuously impinge on children's health and well-being and hamper their education and social development. What has come to be called a "revolution in child health and survival" is possible and practicable today. It would have enormous immediate benefits wherever it was introduced and would not demand an unrealistic reallocation of resources. It would have even greater long-term benefits for the health, well-being, and development of all societies.

Targeting services and support to those most in need

Each national, city, and local government authority must identify the groups in its jurisdiction that are most in need of services and support. Each authority must design and implement action geared to the particular health and housing problems of the people within its jurisdiction. Infants and children will figure prominently as those most in need of special measures and programmes in virtually all instances. National and provincial government authorities seeking to make the best use of limited resources for improving health, and to target help to those most in need, should note that generalizations about "rural" versus "urban" are usually inaccurate. First, such generalizations obscure the often enormous variations between urban centres in the quality of their public services. This is also true of rural districts. Certainly, the inhabitants of many small and intermediate-size urban centres have no better access to public health services and to protected water supplies than rural inhabitants have. Secondly, as figures given earlier have shown, the lower income groups in the largest cities can have levels of infant and child mortality and ill health comparable with those found in the poorer rural groups. While the majority of the inhabitants of developing countries live in rural areas, there are over a thousand million urban dwellers in the Third World and of these, over 500 million are infants and children. In addition, many countries and regions are predominantly urban — for instance, nearly three-quarters of the population of Latin America lives in urban areas. In the Caribbean area, East Asia (other than China), and Western Asia, more than half the population lives in urban areas.

The process of identifying the groups with the most serious health problems and those not reached by public services and facilities is likely to show that these correlate more closely with such factors as low and unstable incomes, specific high-risk occupations, age (especially in the case of infants and children), and gender than with whether the people concerned live in "rural" or "urban" areas. National capitals and large cities usually have a high concentration of the countries' hospital beds, physicians, and water supply and sanitation facilities, but this does not mean that the poorest 30–60% of the population in these cities benefit from them.

Coordination of action

Effective action demands coordinated programmes from different sectoral agencies and at different levels of government. Table 8 summarizes the different types of action needed at individual and household level, at neighbourhood and community level, at city and district level, and at national level. It gives an idea of the wide range of factors that influence each individual's state of health. It also shows the number of government agencies or ministries whose policies and programmes can, and should, promote better health.

With limited resources, public health agencies alone can achieve only limited results in terms of both prevention and cure. For instance, improvement in the treatment of childhood diarrhoea (the world's most common childhood disease and the leading cause of

Table 8. Links between health and government action at different levels to improve housing conditions in urban residential areas[a]

Health risk	Action at individual and household level	Public action at neighbourhood or community level	Action at city or district level	Action at national level
Contaminated water – typhoid, hepatitis, dysenteries, diarrhoea, cholera, etc.	Protection of water supply to house; promotion of knowledge of hygienic water storage	Provision of water supply infrastructure; promotion of knowledge and motivation in community	Plans to undertake action described and resources to do so	Ensuring that local and city authorities have the power, funding base, and trained personnel to implement action at household, neighbourhood, city and district level; reviewing and, where appropriate, changing legislative framework and norms and codes to allow and encourage action at lower levels and ensure that infrastructure standards are appropriate to needs and available resources; support for training courses and seminars for architects, planners, engineers, etc. on the health aspects of their work
Inadequate disposal of human wastes – pathogens from excreta contaminating food, water, or fingers, leading to faecal–oral transmission of diseases or intestinal worms (e.g. hookworm, tapeworm, roundworm, schistosomiasis)	Support for construction of easily maintained latrine/WC matching physical conditions, social preferences, and economic resources; washing facilities; promotion of hand-washing	Mix of technical advice and installation, servicing, and maintenance of equipment (mix dependent on technology used)	Plans to undertake action described plus resources; ensuring availability of trained personnel and finance for servicing and maintenance	
Waste water and garbage – water-logged soil ideal for transmitting diseases like hookworm; pools of standing water becoming contaminated, conveying enteric diseases and providing breeding ground for mosquitos spreading filariasis, malaria, and other diseases; garbage attracting disease vectors	Provision of storm/surface-water drains and spaces for storing garbage that are ratproof, catproof, dogproof, and childproof	Design and provision of storm/ surface-water drains; advice to households on materials and construction techniques to make houses less damp	Regular removal, or provision for safe disposal, of household wastes; organization of framework and resources for drains	
Insufficient water, facilities for washing and for personal hygiene – ear and eye infections (including trachoma), skin diseases, scabies, lice, fleas	Adequate water supply for washing and bathing; provision for laundry at household or community level	Health and personal hygiene education for children and adults; facilities for laundry at this level, if not within individual houses	Support for health education and public facilities for laundry	Technical and financial support for educational campaigns; coordination of housing, health, and education ministries
Disease vectors or parasites in house structure with access to occupants/food/water, e.g. rats, cockroaches, and other insects (including vector of Chagas' disease)	Support for improved house structure – e.g., tiled floors, protected food-storage areas, roofs/walls/floors protected from disease vectors	Technical advice and information as part of adult/child education programme	Loans for upgrading house; guaranteed supply of cheap and easily available materials, fixtures, and fittings	Ensuring that building codes and official procedures to approve house construction/improvement are not inhibiting individual, household, and local government action; support for nationwide availability of building loans, cheap materials (where possible based on local resources), and building-advice centres; production of technical and educational material in this connection
Inadequate house size/ventilation – helps spread diseases such as tuberculosis, influenza and meningitis (aerosol drop transmission) and increases frequency of diseases transmitted through interhuman contact (e.g. mumps and measles); risks of household accidents increased with overcrowding; it becomes impossible to safeguard children from poisons and open fires or stoves	Technical advice and financial support for house improvement or extension, and provision of cheap sites with basic services in different parts of the city to offer low-income groups alternatives to their current shelter	Technical advice on improving ventilation; education on diseases and accidents related to overcrowding	Loans (including small ones with flexible repayment); support for building-advice centres in each neighbourhood	

SUMMARY, CONCLUSIONS, AND RECOMMENDATIONS

Health problem	Household-level action	Community-level action	Municipal/city-level action	National-level action
Children playing in and around house constantly exposed to dangers from traffic, unsafe sites, or sites contaminated with faeces or pollutants	Organization of child care services to look after children in households where all adults work	Provision within each neighbourhood of well-drained site separated from traffic, kept clean and free from garbage, easily supervised and with first-aid services close to hand	Support for neighbourhood-level play, sport, and recreation facilities.	National legislation and financial and technical support for interventions by local and city governments in land markets to support lower-level action; getting training institutions to provide needed personnel at each level
Indoor air pollution through open fires or poorly designed stoves exacerbates respiratory illness, especially in women and children	Posters/booklets or improved stove design and improving ventilation, etc.	Ensuring availability of designs and materials for improved models; investigating possibilities of promoting use of alternative fuels		
House sites subject to landslides or floods as result of no other land being affordable to lower-income groups	Regularization of each household's tenure if dangers can be lessened; relocation through offer of alternative sites	Action to reduce dangers and encourage upgrading or offer of alternative sites	Ensuring availability of safe housing sites that lower income groups can afford	
Illegal occupation of house site or illegal subdivision with disincentive to upgrade, lack of services, and mental stress from fear of eviction	Regularization of each household's tenure and provision for piped water, sanitation, and storm and surface-water drainage	Local government working with community to provide basic infrastructure and services and incorporation into "official city"	Support for incorporating illegal subdivisions and for providing tenure to squatter households	
Nutritional deficiencies and low income	Action to reduce worm burden and worm transmission support for income-generating work within the house	Food supplements/school meals; support for enterprises in low-income settlements or set up by their inhabitants; if land is available, promote its use for growing vegetables; if malnutrition is serious, consider most appropriate programme to reach most seriously affected groups		Structural reforms, funds for food supplementation or other emergency nutrition programmes, and other measures to improve poorer groups' real income
No or inadequate access to curative/preventive health care and advice	Widespread availability of simple primer on first aid and health in the home with home visits by health workers to promote its use	Primary health care centre; emphasis on child and maternal health, preventive health, and support for community action and for community volunteers	Small hospital (first referral level) and resources and training to support lower level services and volunteers	Technical and financial support for nationwide system of hospitals and health care centres; preventive health campaigns (e.g., immunization) and nationwide availability of drugs and equipment; setting-up training system for auxiliary/community health workers; provision of guidelines for setting up emergency services and planning and risk minimization in risk-prone areas to limit injuries and damage if disaster occurs
No provision for emergency life-saving services in event of injury or serious illness	Widespread availability of simple primer on first aid and health in the home with educational programmes on minimizing risks	Basic equipment (e.g. stretchers, first aid kit) available and accessible 24 hours a day; community volunteer's with basic training on call and arrangements for rapid transfer of sick person to hospital; equipment to rescue and treat people saved from burning houses	Support for neighbourhood-level equipment, plus organization of training programmes for community volunteers; fire-fighting equipment; contingency plans for emergencies	
	Discussions with individuals and community organizations about some minimum changes in site layout to improve emergency access of vehicles and create fire breaks			

[a] Source: HARDOY, J. E. & SATTERTHWAITE, D. Housing and health: do architects and planners have a role? *Cities*, **4**, 221–235 (1987). Many of the above measures to improve the quality of the services and facilities a house contains will often have to be modified in the case of houses, flats, rooms, or house sites that are rented. A high proportion of the lowest-income individuals and households in most Third World cities rent their accommodation, and improving its quality and reducing the health risks it presents will need government programmes and action that are not summarized in this table.

death in childhood) can have little impact if nothing is done at the same time to reduce the risk of reinfection (for instance, campaigns to promote breast-feeding and to put pressure on national agencies and local government authorities to install potable piped-water supplies and to ensure the hygienic removal of household and human wastes). Even if action is taken on all these fronts, the effects will still be limited if most children remain seriously undernourished, so a programme to tackle malnutrition in children would be needed. This too would need to be coordinated with action by agencies other than those directly concerned with health.

Coordinated action at different levels between different sectors of government can make the best use of limited resources. The present economic crisis prevents most governments in developing countries from improving the living conditions of the urban poor in the conventional manner (e.g., by providing piped water and sewers for each house, paved roads, sidewalks, drainage, electricity, and health care, preventive, and emergency life-saving services of a standard similar to that found in developed countries). But there are innovative approaches that can significantly improve health and well-being at far lower cost. These approaches require coordinated multi-sectoral action by public agencies at national and local level. They require architects, planners, engineers, and all agencies with some role in designing, planning, building, or maintaining the man-made environment to become aware of all they can do to improve the health of people in lower income groups, and of how their action can help reduce threats to health. Finally, they often imply public action defined, coordinated, and assisted by neighbourhood associations.

The key to cost-effectiveness often lies in new partnerships with community or neighbourhood organizations. Mention was made in earlier chapters of the active community organizations formed by groups of urban residents. Many more would be formed, or would be more effective, if they received financial support and technical assistance from government agencies. A key change in government thinking would be to recognize that, to date, public housing programmes have done little to improve living conditions for lower-income groups, that these groups are already building most of the new housing, and that the public authorities must modify all the norms, codes, and standards to support and assist their efforts. Instead of demanding structural standards and the use of building materials that few households can afford, they must provide advice centres that will promote the attainment of health and safety standards at minimum cost. Instead of mounting costly surveys to determine health problems, they must work with neighbourhood associations to identify the most pressing problems and act on them. Instead of feeling unable to start installing sewerage and storm drainage systems in existing squatter communities, because it would cost too much, they must review with neighbourhood associations the possibility of interim measures to deal with the most serious problems.

Neighbourhood organizations and their federations can become a powerful and effective force in tackling environmental health problems. The right kind of support and technical assistance from municipal and city authorities, nongovernmental bodies (e.g., research or professional groups), and aid agencies can greatly increase their effectiveness.

Community or neighbourhood organizations and federations are generally more active wherever city and municipal authorities are elected and resources to deal with environmental health problems are readily forthcoming. Neighbourhood organizations can set priorities and join with local authorities and nongovernmental organizations in surveys to identify the main health problems and the action needed to deal with them in the shape of environmental improvements and preventive measures (*96*). This can mean major savings in time and money. For instance, if access roads are to be introduced into squatter settlements, and this means that some houses have to be moved, the whole neighbourhood may be strongly opposed to the scheme. But the full involvement of neighbourhood organizations in determining priorities for health improvement — including the introduction of access roads — has been shown to minimize opposition to the measures proposed. In some cases, the professional staff taking part have recognized that neighbourhood organizations have actually improved on their site plans.

This alliance between neighbourhood-based organizations, local and national nongovernmental organizations, and local government authorities can be a most powerful and cost-effective force for the improvement of environmental health. Experience has shown that such an alliance is effective only if the authorities at the neighbourhood, city, and national levels can provide the needed support and guidance. Members of low-income households generally have very limited amounts of free time to devote to communal activities; even those who are registered as "unemployed" or "underemployed", are likely to work long hours, 6 or 7 days a week. They will not devote time and energy to environmental improvements unless they can be assured of genuine results.

The key role of local government

Local government should be responsible for planning and coordinating action by sectoral ministries or agencies (for instance, building roads, providing health care services, installing potable water supplies, etc.) within their area of jurisdiction. However, local government authorities are often so weak and ineffective that they have virtually no capacity for investment in infrastructure and are not equipped to coordinate the work of national agencies within their jurisdiction. Local government action must also respond to and support the demands of organized groups representing low-income communities. Local government officials may then succeed in becoming the main intermediaries between community organizations and the central and/or state government. Local government authorities must have the power and resources to ensure that the most urgent public interventions at the local level, such as the provision of basic infrastructure and services, cheap legal land sites for new low-income housing, and technical advice on improving housing conditions, will represent a direct or indirect improvement in the health and safety of the local inhabitants. It is thus important to strengthen local government, reversing the general trend observed in almost all developing countries in recent decades.

The role of nongovernmental organizations

In many developing countries nongovernmental organizations have an important role as originators, agents, and supporters of new approaches to the task of improving the health and housing of lower-income groups, and as technical and legal advisors to community organizations. In many urban centres, neither the local authority nor the international aid agencies working there have even begun to tap their potential as intermediaries between the national or state government and community organizations in the upgrading of improvement schemes (53). Nongovernmental organizations have often proved particularly skilled and sympathetic in work with specific disadvantaged groups such as street children with limited or no contact with their families, the homeless, and the permanently disabled.

National government

Governments must build up or strengthen legal and institutional structures to facilitate the implementation of the multisectoral measures described above. The responsibility of the national government is not so much to provide basic amenities, improve nutritional levels, and organize basic preventive health, health care, and emergency life-saving services, as to build up the legal and institutional structures of government at city and district level to permit urban authorities to carry out these tasks; and to ensure that the authorities have access to the trained personnel, capital and revenue required for this purpose, and for the necessary basic urban infrastructure.

SUMMARY, CONCLUSIONS, AND RECOMMENDATIONS

The implementation of the measures just noted would require the allocation of a higher proportion of resources to the improvement of living conditions and the provision of basic services than that allocated today by most national governments. These activities are currently given low priority at the national level and hence a low proportion of public funds. While very few cities or countries have the resources to follow "western" precedents in this area, virtually all of them can achieve real improvements in their citizens' health and housing by following the approach outlined here.

Three critical areas for national governments are: increased funding for water, sanitation, and drainage; increased funding for preventive health measures and primary health care; and increased action to control pollution. As already noted, it is possible, at relatively low cost, greatly to increase the number of households with access to safe and sufficient supplies of water. Indeed, the per capita cost for new systems can often be fully recovered by charges to the users, which would still be lower than the sums currently paid to water-vendors for inadequate and sometimes unsafe water by people in low-income groups. There are systems for the collection of human wastes, and for the removal of wastewater and storm and surface run-off, that are far cheaper than conventional sewerage and storm drainage systems. As has been shown, costs can be reduced very considerably if government agencies work in liaison with community organizations. A combination of safe and sufficient water supply, sanitation, and storm drainage can greatly improve child health and reduce infant and child mortality. When this is combined with preventive programmes (especially immunization to protect children from measles, poliomyelitis, tuberculosis, diptheria, tetanus, and pertussis) and the provision of health care and emergency services, the chances of child survival can be multiplied many times. The reduction in the toll exacted by disease and accidents can be as dramatic. For more prosperous developing countries, a 5–10 year programme that will greatly increase the proportion of people reached by the requisite improvements is affordable. In the poorer countries, much could be achieved through the better use of existing resources, although external funding will be needed.

Action to control pollution can also bring about major health benefits. In many countries, urgent action is needed to reduce the exposure of children to airborne lead emitted by factories and internal combustion engines, and to lead from other sources (for instance, lead-based paints). In many cities, governments must act to limit emissions of nitrogen and sulfur oxides and particulate matter, as this would bring major health benefits, notably a reduction in the incidence of respiratory diseases. The high rate of respiratory diseases in the Third World and the serious risk they present for young children of poor families was noted in an earlier chapter. In many instances, government action is needed to help low-income groups use fuels or stoves of a type that will reduce health-damaging emissions within the home and in the wider city environment.

Aid agencies

Virtually all aid agencies acknowledge that support for activities of the kind outlined above is important, effective, and cost-effective. But few of them give high priority to such activities when allocating funds. Inevitably, there are operational difficulties in giving higher priority to projects and programmes that bring immediate health benefits to the poorer urban groups. One of these difficulties is the inevitable increase in staff time; large civic construction projects are much easier and cheaper to supervise. A second is the reluctance of recipient governments to give high priority to health-promoting projects in negotiations with donors. Aid agencies could overcome both these difficulties by channelling more funds to water supply, sanitation, and drainage schemes, the production of cheap building materials, credits for building or improving housing, preventive activities, and primary health care, through nongovernmental organizations and private voluntary agencies from developed countries that are already working in low-income communities in the Third World. Another option would be for each aid agency to set aside a proportion of its funds whose allocation and use would be supervised by a special multidisciplinary team dedicated to the promotion of child health and survival. Third World governments respond to what they see as priorities of external support agencies, and such a move would encourage these governments to pay more attention to activities in this area.

The aid agencies have a responsibility to initiate urgent action now. Their collective example could do much to set the requisite measures in motion throughout the Third World. Of course, such measures are not the whole solution. Poverty and ill health in developing countries are as much the result of deeply rooted inequalities in income and power at the world level as they are at the national level. Problems such as street children, widespread malnutrition, or growing squatter settlements can be permanently solved only when the vast majority of the world's people either own enough agricultural land, or earn sufficiently well to afford enough food to satisfy their hunger and their nutritional needs, and to build, buy, or rent an adequate house with piped water and sanitation without having to work excessive hours and rely on children's earnings for survival. Nevertheless, the approach recommended here could reduce much of the burden of ill health, disablement, and premature death that weighs on hundreds of millions of urban children in the

Third World today. Such an approach could make a major contribution to the achievement of health for all by the year 2000.

The success with which societies deal with deprivation in childhood and its attendant problems has major implications for their future development. The future development of societies in the Third World will be considerably influenced by the daily experiences of their children and by the opportunities provided for them today. A society cannot realize its potential for economic advancement or achieve a socially concerned, democratic government as long as a high proportion of its citizens have had childhoods characterized by poverty and deprivation, with the result that many of them are permanently impaired or disabled by malnutrition, disease, and accidents that could have been prevented.

References

1. ACHAYO WERE P. T. The development of road transport in Africa and its effects on land use and environment. *Industry and environment*, **6** (2): 25–26 (1983).
2. AGARWAL, D. K., ET AL. Morbidity pattern in underfive children. *Journal of tropical pediatrics*, **28**: 139–143 (1982).
3. ALVAREZ, M. DE LA LUZ ET AL. Caracteristicas de familias urbanas con lactante desnutrido. *Archivos latino-americanos de nutrición*, **29** (2): 220–232 (1979).
4. ANGEL, S. ET AL., ed. *Land for housing the poor*. Singapore, Select Books, 1983.
5. Another development in health (report on Dag Hammerskjold seminar, 1977). *Development dialogue (Uppsala)*, (1978).
6. BALLESTEROS, G. M. ET AL. Concentración de plomo en sangre de niños de familias alfareras. *Boletín de la Oficina Sanitaria Panamericana*, **92** (1): 33–40 (1982).
7. BAPAT, M. & CROOK, N. The environment, health and nutrition: an analysis of interrelationships from a case study of hutment settlements in the city of Poona. *Habitat international*, 8 (3/4): 115–126 (1984).
8. BARILOCHE FOUNDATION. *Catastrophe or new society?* Ottawa, International Development Resources Centre, 1977.
9. BASTA, S. S. Nutrition and health in low-income urban areas of the Third World. *Ecology of food and nutrition* **6**: 113–124 (1977).
10. BERNAL, M. E. & ULPIANO, A. Child labour in Bogotá. In: Carrion, D & Vainstoc, A., ed., *La ciudad y los niños*. Quito, Editorial El Conejo-CIUDAD, 1987.
11. BISHARAT, L. & TEWFIK, M. Housing the urban poor in Amman. Can upgrading improve health? *Third World planning review*, **7** (1): 5–22 (1985).
12. BLITZER, S. ET AL. The sectoral and spatial distribution of multilateral aid for human settlements. *Habitat international*, **7** (1/2): 103–127 (1983).
13. BRASILEIRO, A. M. ET AL. Extending municipal services by building on local initiatives—a project in the favelas of Rio de Janeiro. *Assignment children*, **57/58**: 66–100 (1982).
14. BRISCOE, J. Water supply and health in developing countries: selective primary health care revisited. In: Tulchin, J. S., ed., *Habitat, health and development*. Boulder, CO, Lynne Rienner, 1986, pp. 105–124.
15. BRUCE-CHWATT, L. J. Paludisme et urbanisation. *Bulletin de la Societé de Pathologie Exotique*, **76**: 243–249 (1983).
16. CARROLL, A. *Pirate subdivisions and the market for residential lots in Bogotá.* Washington, DC, World Bank, 1980 (World Bank Staff Working Paper No. 435).
17. Carta economica. *Diario el cronista comercial*, Buenos Aires, December 1985.
18. CARVALHO, F. M. ET AL. Lead poisoning among children from Santo Amaro, Brazil. *Bulletin of the Pan American Health Organization*, **19** (2): 165–175 (1985).
19. CHAUHAN, S. K. *Who puts the water in the taps?* London, Earthscan, 1983.

20. *Child abuse and urban slum environments. WHO/ISPCAN pre-congress workshop.* Unpublished WHO document, WHO/MCH/86.15. (A limited number of copies are available on request from Maternal and Child Health, World Health Organization, 1211 Geneva 27, Switzerland.)

21. CHISHOLM, J. J. Removal of lead paint from old housing: the need for a new approach. *American journal of public health*, **76** (3): 236–237 (1986).

22. CHOSSUDOWSKY, M. Atención primaria y sanitaria en América Latina. In: *Pobreza, necesidades basicas y desarrollo*, Santiago, Chile, CEPAL/ILPES/UNICEF, 1982.

23. COCHRANE, G. *Policies for strengthening local government in developing countries.* Washington, DC, World Bank, 1983 (World Bank Staff Working Paper No. 582), p. 5.

24. CUENYA, B. ET AL. *Condiciones de habitat y salud de los sectores populares: un estudio piloto.* Buenos Aires, Ediciones CEUR, 1984.

25. DA SILVA, L. J. Crecimento urbano e doenca. A equistossomose no município de São Paulo. *Revista saude publica (São Paulo)*, **19**: 1–7 (1985).

26. DATTA-BANIK, N. D. Some observations on feeding programmes, nutrition and growth of preschool children in an urban community. *Indian journal of pediatrics*, **44**: 139–149 (1977).

27. DATTA-BANIK, N. D. Feeding habits and weaning practices in infants and preschool children in slum areas of New Delhi. *Archives of child health*, **21** (3): 51–57 (1979).

28. DONOHUE, J. Some facts and figures on urbanization in the developing world. *Assignment children*, **57–58**: 21–41 (1982).

29. ELMENDORF, M. L. & ISELY, R. B. Role of women in water supply and sanitation. *World health forum*, **3** (2): 227–230 (1982).

30. GILBERT, A. Pirates and invaders: Land acquisition in urban Colombia and Venezuela. *World development*, **9**: 657–678 (1981).

31. GONZÁLEZ, L. U. & ZÚÑIGA, D. C. Costumbres sobre saneamiento básico en población suburbana. Estudio de Viña del Mar. *Boletín de la Oficina Sanitaria Panamericana*, **94** (5): 482–494 (1983).

32. GUBER, R. Villas miseria: la organización informal del espacio urbano. *Boletín del medio ambiente y urbanización*, Year 2 (5): 39–42 (1983).

33. HAMZA, A. Management of industrial hazardous wastes in Egypt. In: *Industry and environment.* Paris, United Nations Environment Programme, 1983.

34. HARDOY, J. E. The inhabitants of historical centres: who is concerned about their plight? *Habitat international*, **7** (5/6): 151–162 (1983).

35. HARDOY, J. E. & DOS SANTOS, M. *Impacto de la urbanización en los centros historicos latinamericanos.* Lima, UNDP/UNESCO, 1982.

36. HARDOY, J. E. & SATTERTHWAITE, D. Shelter, infrastructure and services in Third World cities. *Habitat international*, **10** (3/4): 245–284 (1986).

37. HARDOY, J. E. & SATTERTHWAITE, D., ed. *Small and intermediate urban centres: their role in regional and national development in the Third World.* London, Hodder & Stoughton and New York, Westview, 1986.

38. HARDOY, J. E. & SATTERTHWAITE, D. Third World cities and the environment of poverty. *Geoforum*, **15** (3): 307–333 (1984).

39. HARDOY, J. E. & SATTERTHWAITE, D. Housing and health: do architects and planners have a role? *Cities*, **4**: 221–235 (1987).

40. *Hechos urbanos. Boletin de información y analisis*, 21–34. Santiago de Chile, SUR Documentación, 1983–85.

41. HINKLE, L. E. & LORING, W. C., ed. *The effect of the man-made environment on health and behaviour*. Washington, DC, Center for Disease Control, Public Health Service, US Department of Health, Education and Welfare, 1977.

42. HOGE, W. New menace in Brazil's valley of death strikes unborn. *New York Times*, 25 September 1980.

43. HORN, J. The medical brain drain and health priorities in Latin America. *International journal of health services*, 7: 425–442 (1977).

44. JACOBI, P. Movimentos populares urbanos e resposta do estado: autonomia e controle vs. cooptaçao e clintelismo. In: Boschi, R., ed. *Movimentos coletivos no Brasil urbano*. Rio de Janeiro, Zahar Ed., 1983 (Debates Urbanos 5).

45. KALBERMATTEN, J. M. ET AL. *Appropriate technology for water supply and sanitation: a review of the technical and economic options*. Washington, DC, World Bank, 1980.

46. KEREJAN, H. & N'DA KONAN. Approches des problemes alimentaires et nutritionnels d'une megalopolis africaine. *Médecin Afrique noire*, **28** (7): 479–482 (1981).

47. KEYES, W. J. Metro-Manila, Philippines. In: Sahrin, M., ed., *Policies towards urban slums*. Bangkok, Economic and Social Commission for Asia and the Pacific, 1980.

48. KOTHARI, G. ET AL. Appraisal of current conditions of health in Greater Bombay. Paper presented at the *Seminar on Problems of Public Health in Metropolitan Cities, with particular reference to Greater Bombay, 8–9 March 1983*. Bombay, International Institute for Population Studies, 1983.

49. LARREA, C. M. Crecimiento urbano y dinamica de las ciudades intermedias en el Ecuador. In: Carrion, D. et al., ed., *Ciudades en conflicto*, Quito, Editorial El Conejo-CIUDAD, 1986, pp. 89–126.

50. LEE, J. A. *The environment, public health and human ecology*. Baltimore and London, Johns Hopkins University, 1985.

51. LEONARD, H. J. *Confronting industrial pollution in rapidly industrializing countries: myths, pitfalls and opportunities*. Washington, DC, Conservation Foundation, 1984.

52. LEWIS, C. & LEWIS, M. A. Improving the health of the children: must the children be involved?. *Annual review of public health*, 4: 259–283 (1983).

53. *Limuru declaration, working principles and recommendations*. Paper produced by participants in the Seminar on Non-Government Organizations; their Role in Shelter, Services and Community Development, held at Limuru, Kenya, in April 1987. Settlements information network Africa, Newsletter No. 14, July 1987.

54. LINDHEIM, R. Environment, people and health. *Annual review of public health*, 4: 335–359 (1983).

55. MAHAFFEY, K. R. ET AL. National estimates of blood lead levels: United States, 1976–1980. Association with selected demographic and socioeconomic factors. *New England journal of medicine*, **307**: 573–579 (1982).

56. MARTIN, A. E., ed. *Health aspects of human settlements*. Geneva, World Health Organization, 1977 (Public Health Paper, No. 66).

57. MCAUSLAN, P. *Urban land and shelter for the poor*. London and Washington, DC, Earthscan, 1985.

58. Ministry of Public Health and Social Services of El Salvador and Nutrition Institute of Central America and Panama (INCAP). *Clasificación funcional de*

problemas nutricionales en El Salvador. Informe final. Guatemala, INCAP, 1977.

59. MISRA, H. N. *Popular settlements in the city of Allahabad (India) and the health problems of their inhabitants: findings from three case studies.* Allahabad, International Institute for Development Research, 1987.

60. MOSER, C. O. N. *Housing policy and women: towards a gender-aware approach.* London, University College, 1984 (DPU Gender and Planning Working Paper).

61. MOSER, C. O. N. *Residential level struggle and consciousness: the experience of poor women in Guayaquil, Ecuador.* London, University College, 1985 (DPU Gender and Planning Working Paper).

62. National Institute of Natural Resources and the Environment (IRENA). *Taller internacional de salvamento y aprovechamiento integral del Lago de Managua, 2.* Managua, 1982.

63. NATIONAL NUTRITION INSTITUTE. *Survey 1963-1965.* Bogotá, Government of Colombia.

64. NEEDLEMAN, H. The health effects of low level exposure to lead. *Annual review of public health,* **2**: 277-298, (1981).

65. NJAU, G. Human settlements in the 1980s: Nairobi's experience. In: Blair, T., ed., *Papers and proceedings of Habitat Forum Conference.* London, Polytechnic of Central London, 1982.

66. Nutritional surveillance. Global trends in protein-energy-malnutrition prevalence. *Weekly epidemiological record,* **59** (25): 188-192 (1984).

67. PASTERNAK, S. Las favelas del muncipio de San Pablo. Resultados de una investigación. *Revista interamericana de planificación,* **14**: 50-67 (1980).

68. PIO, A. ET AL. Bases for WHO Programme on Acute Respiratory Infections (ARI) in children. *Bulletin of the International Union Against Tuberculosis,* **58**: 199-208 (1983).

69. PIO, A. ET AL. *The magnitude of the problem of acute respiratory infections in children. Proceedings of an international workshop, Sydney, 1984.* University of Adelaide, 1985, pp. 3-16.

70. POPULATION CRISIS COMMITTEE. *World population growth and global security.,* 1983 (Briefing Paper No. 13).

71. *Primary health care. Report of the International Conference on Primary Health Care, Alma-Ata, USSR, 6-12 September 1978.* Geneva, World Health Organization, 1978.

72. Principales problemas ambientales de América Latina. *Boletín de la Oficina Sanitaria Panamericana,* **94** (4): 410-416 (1983).

73. PUFFER, R. R. & SERRANO, C. V. *Patterns of mortality in childhood.* Washington, DC, Pan American Health Organization, 1973 (Scientific Publication No. 262).

74. RICE, C. Behavioural deficit (delaying matching to sample) in monkeys exposed from birth to low levels of lead. *Toxicology and applied pharmacology* **75**: 337-345 (1984).

75. RIVAS, E. *Estudio analítico de un submercado de vivienda: arrendamiento de piezas* (informe final de investigación). Buenos Aires, CEUR-ITDT, 1977.

76. RODHE, J. E. Why the other half dies: the science and politics of child mortality in the Third World. *Assignment children,* **61–62**: 35-37 (1983)

77. RODRIGUEZ, A. Notas para el analisis del suburbio y tugurio de Guayaquil *Revista interamericana de planificación,* **14**: 151-159 (1980).

78. RUTTER, M. Low-level lead exposures: sources, effects and implications. In: Rutter, M. & Jones, R. R., ed. *Lead versus health; sources and effects of low-level*

lead exposure. Chichester and New York, John Wiley and Sons, 1982, pp. 333–370.

79. SANTANA, P. La crisis urbana y el poder local y regional; el case Colombiano. In: Carrion, D. et al., ed, *Ciudades en conflicto*, Quito Editorial El Conejo-CIUDAD, 1986, pp. 283–300.

79a. SHRIVASTAV, P. P. City for the citizen or citizen for the city; the search for an appropriate strategy for slums and housing the urban poor in developing countries — the case of Delhi. *Habitat international*, **6**: 197–207 (1982).

80. SIGULEM, D. M. & TUDISCO, E. S. Aleitamento natural em diferentes classes de renda no municipio de São Paulo. *Archivos latino-americanos de nutrición*, **30** (3): 400–416 (1980).

81. SINGER, P. Movimentos de barrio. In: Singer, P. & Caldeira Brant, V., ed., *São Paulo: o povo em movimento*. Rio de Janeiro, Ed. VOZ es-CEBRAP, 1980.

82. SMIL, V. *The bad earth: environmental degradation in China*. New York, M. E. Sharpe and London, Zed Press, 1984.

83. SNYDER, J. D. & MERSON, M. H. The magnitude of the global problem of acute diarrhoeal disease: a review of active surveillance data. *Bulletin of the World Health Organization*, **60** (4): 605–613 (1982).

84. *State of India's environment 1982: a citizen's report*. Delhi, Centre for Science and Environment, 1983.

85. *State of India's environment 1984–85: a second citizen's report*. Delhi, Centre for Science and Environment, 1986.

86. *The city — a nightmare for children*. Supplement to *Hoy* newspaper, Quito, 1987.

87. THEUNYNCK, S. DIA, M. The young (and the less young) in infra-urban areas in Mauritania. *African environment*, **14, 15, 16**: (1981).

88. TULCHIN, J. S., ed. *Habitat, health, and development. A new way of looking at cities in the Third World*. Boulder, CO, Lynne Rienner, 1986.

89. TURNER, J. F. C. *Housing by people. Ideas in progress*. London, Marion Boyars, 1976.

90. UNITED NATIONS CENTRE FOR HUMAN SETTLEMENTS (HABITAT). *The role of small and intermediate settlements in national development*. Nairobi, 1985.

90a. UNITED NATIONS POPULATION DIVISION. World population prospects, estimates and projections as assessed in 1982. New York, United Nations, 1985 (Population studies, No. 86).

91. URIBE, L. J. The problem of *Aedes aegypti* control in the Americas. *Bulletin of the Pan American Health Organization*, **17** (2): 133–141 (1983).

92. URIBE, L. J. ET AL. Experimental aerial spraying with ultra-low-volume (ULV) malathion to control *Aedes aegypti* in Buga, Colombia. *Bulletin of the Pan American Health Organization*, **18** (1): 43–57 (1984).

93. VINOCUR, P. Clasificación funcional de poblaciones desnutridas en Costa Rica. *Boletín informativo de S.I.N.*, 2 February 1980.

94. WARD, P. M., ed. *Self-help housing: a critique*. London, Mansell, 1982.

95. WHO Technical Report Series, No. 639, 1979 (*Human viruses in water, wastewater and soil*: report of a WHO Scientific Group).

96. WORLD HEALTH ORGANIZATION. *Improving environmental health conditions in low-income settlements*. Geneva, 1987 (WHO Offset Publication, No. 100).

97. WORLD HEALTH ORGANIZATION. *Health principles of housing*. Geneva, 1989.

98. ZICCARDI, A. Formas organizativas de los asentamientos humanos marginados y politica estatal. *Revista interamericana de planificación*, **14** (54): 28–40 (1980).

Annex 1
WHO/UNEP Technical Panel on Environmental Health Aspects of Housing and Urban Planning
Moscow, USSR, 18–24 April 1985

List of participants
Members*

Professor H. L. Cohen, Department of Design Studies, School of Architecture and Environmental Design, State University of New York at Buffalo, NY, USA

Dr L. Dorich, President, National Institute of Urban Development, Ministry of Housing and Construction, Lima, Peru (*Vice-Chairman*)

Dr G. Goldstein, School of Public Health and Tropical Medicine, Sydney University, Sydney, Australia (*Chairman*)

Dr Y. A. Hassan, Assistant Under-Secretary, Ministry of Construction and Public Works, Khartoum, Sudan

Miss H. Vanlankveld-Kiwasila, Ministry of Lands, Natural Resources and Tourism, Sewerage and Drainage, Dar es Salaam, United Republic of Tanzania

Dr F. Kloutse, Deputy Director, National Environmental Health Service, Lomé, Togo

Dr N. N. Litvinov, Deputy Director, A. N. Sysin Institute for Research in General and Community Hygiene, Moscow, USSR

Dr J. Mijic-Vuckovic, Director, Research Unit, Public Health Institute, Belgrade, Yugoslavia

Dr E. A. R. Ouano, Consulting Engineer, Makati, Philippines

Dr D. Satterthwaite, Senior Research Associate, Human Settlements Programme, International Institute for Environment and Development, London, England (*Rapporteur*)

Mr H. Suselo, Director of Planning and Programming, Directorate-General for Human Settlements, Jakarta, Indonesia

---

* Unable to attend: Dr W. Hassouna, SINAI Construction Group, Cairo, Egypt; Dr E. Helwa, Director of Environmental Health, Ministry of Health, Cairo, Egypt; Dr P. Khanna, Indian Institute of Technology, Bombay, India

Observers

Dr S. Christyakova, Chief, Microclimate of Settlements, Central Scientific Research and Design Institute of Town Planning of Gosgrazhdanstroy, Moscow, USSR

Dr S. Grigorevskaya, Project Coordinator, Centre for International Projects, State Committee of Science and Technology, Moscow, USSR

Dr J. Gubernsky, Chief, Department of Hygiene of Populated Areas, Planning and Hygiene, Department of Houses and Official Buildings, A. N. Sysin Institute for Research in General and Community Hygiene, Moscow, USSR

Dr I. Karagodina, Head, Laboratory of Environmental Hygiene of Populated Areas, Erisman Hygiene Research Institute, Moscow, USSR

Secretariat

Mr I. Burton, Paris, France (Consultant)

Mr N. Gebremedhin, Environmental Management Service, United Nations Environment Programme, Nairobi, Kenya

Mr R. Novick, Environmental Health in Rural and Urban Development and Housing, World Health Organization, Geneva, Switzerland

WHO publications

ALGERIA: Entreprise nationale du Livre

ARGENTINA: Carlos Hirsch, SRL, Florida 165, Galeri

AUSTRALIA: Hunter Publications, 58A

AUSTRIA: Gerold & Co., Grab

BAHRAIN: United So

BANGLADESH: The WI

BELGIUM: *For books*: Office
Office International des Péri

BHUTAN: *see* India, WHO Regio

BOTSWANA: Botsalo Books (Pty) L

BRAZIL: Centro Latinoamericano de Int
Publicações, C.P. 20381 - Rua Botucatu

BURMA: *see* India, WHO Regional Office

CAMEROON: Cameroon Book Centre, P.O. Bo

CANADA: Canadian Public Health Association, 13
Telex: 21–053–3841)

CHINA: China National Publications Import & Export C

DEMOCRATIC PEOPLE'S REPUBLIC OF KOREA: *see* It

DENMARK: Munksgaard Export and Subscription Service, No

FIJI: The WHO Representative, P.O. Box 113, SUVA

FINLAND: Akateeminen Kirjakauppa, Keskuskatu 2, 00101 HELSINK

FRANCE: Arnette, 2 rue Casimir-Delavigne, 75006 PARIS

GERMAN DEMOCRATIC REPUBLIC: Buchhaus Leipzig, Postfach 140, 7

GERMANY FEDERAL REPUBLIC OF: Govi-Verlag GmbH, Ginnheimerstras   CHBORN — Buch-
handlung Alexander Horn, Kirchgasse 22, Postfach 3340, 6200 WIESBADEN

GREECE: G.C. Eleftheroudakis S.A., Librairie internationale, rue Nikis 4, 105-63 A

HONG KONG: Hong Kong Government Information Services, Publication (Sales) Office   .mation Services Department, No. 1,
Battery Path, Central, HONG KONG.

HUNGARY: Kultura, P.O.B. 149, BUDAPEST 62

ICELAND: Snaebjorn Jonsson & Co., Hafnarstraeti 9, P.O. Box 1131, IS-101 REYKJAVIK

INDIA: WHO Regional Office for South-East Asia, World Health House, Indraprastha Estate, Mahatma Gandhi Road,
NEW DELHI 110002

IRAN (ISLAMIC REPUBLIC OF): Iran University Press, 85 Park Avenue, P.O. Box 54/551, TEHERAN

IRELAND: TDC Publishers, 12 North Frederick Street, DUBLIN 1 (Tel: 744835–749677)

ISRAEL: Heiliger & Co., 3 Nathan Strauss Street, JERUSALEM 94227

ITALY: Edizioni Minerva Medica, Corso Bramante 83–85, 10126 TURIN; Via Lamarmora 3, 20100 MILAN; Via Spallanzani 9,
00161 ROME

JAPAN: Maruzen Co. Ltd., P.O. Box 5050, TOKYO International, 100–31

JORDAN: Jordan Book Centre Co. Ltd., University Street, P.O. Box 301 (Al-Jubeiha), AMMAN

KENYA: Text Book Centre Ltd, P.O. Box 47540, NAIROBI

KUWAIT: The Kuwait Bookshops Co. Ltd., Thunayan Al-Ghanem Bldg, P.O. Box 2942, KUWAIT

LAO PEOPLE'S DEMOCRATIC REPUBLIC: The WHO Representative, P.O. Box 343, VIENTIAN'

LUXEMBOURG: Librairie du Centre, 49 bd Royal, LUXEMBOURG

A/1/88